Abolition of Animal Slavery

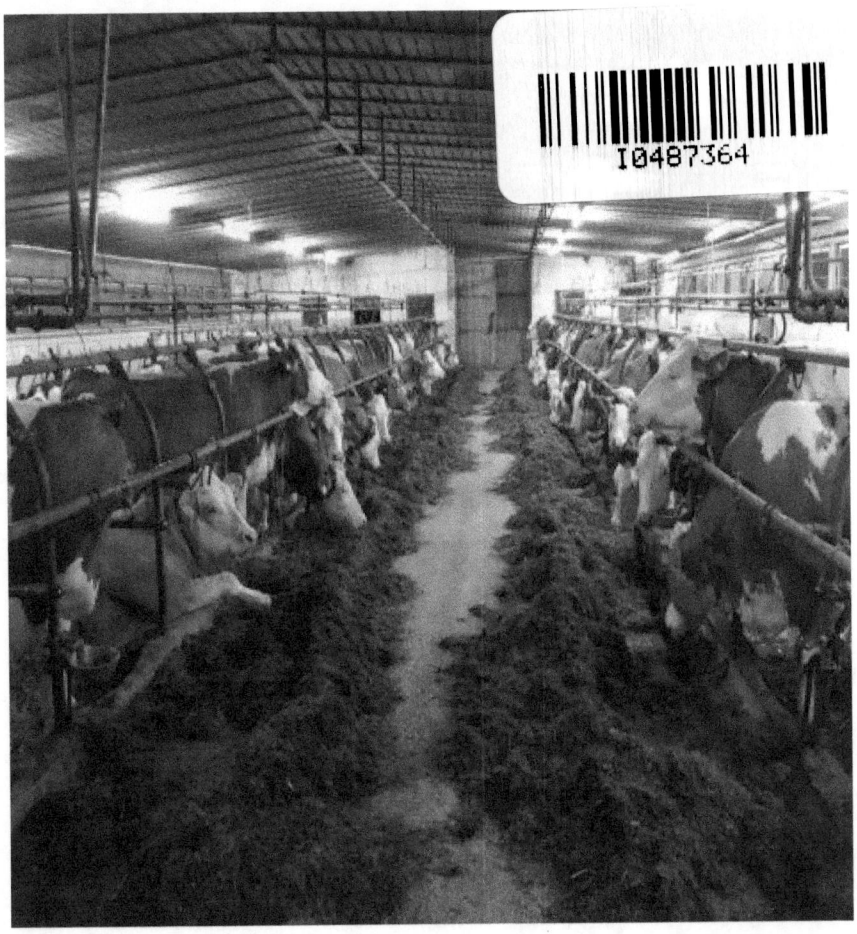

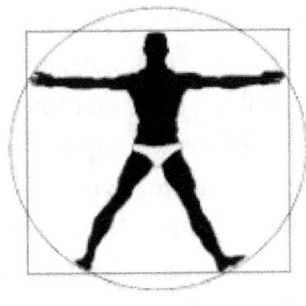

Pigs

Weaning pigs

Rabbits

Dairy cows

Calves

Milk goats

Lambs

Laying hens

Broiler chickens

Pigeons

Civets

Mountain Marmots

Chimpanzees

Dromedaries

Bats

Wildlife

Man and the Animal for Slaughter

Peter A.J. Holst MD PhD

Man takes up all space on earth, both in the circle and in the square, more and more animals are being housed and live only to be eaten by man.

Coronavirus, African Swine Fever, Bovine Leukemia Virus, Avian Leukemia Virus are all uncontrollable phenomena. More than 300 million farm animals in the EU spend their entire life in a cage. The coronavirus pandemic and the worldwide lock down has shown how fragile society really is. Is a pig who suffocates chokingly dead less important than a human who dies chokingly. It is not an animal activist who speaks here, but a doctor who is looking for a solution. Meat and dairy consumption continue to rise worldwide, wiping away wildlands, bringing us into contact with potentially dangerous viruses. The world is turned upside down and our knowledge and insights are increasing rapidly. Stop eating and slaughtering animals and the production of cultured meat will become the solution for climate change and emerging pandemics.

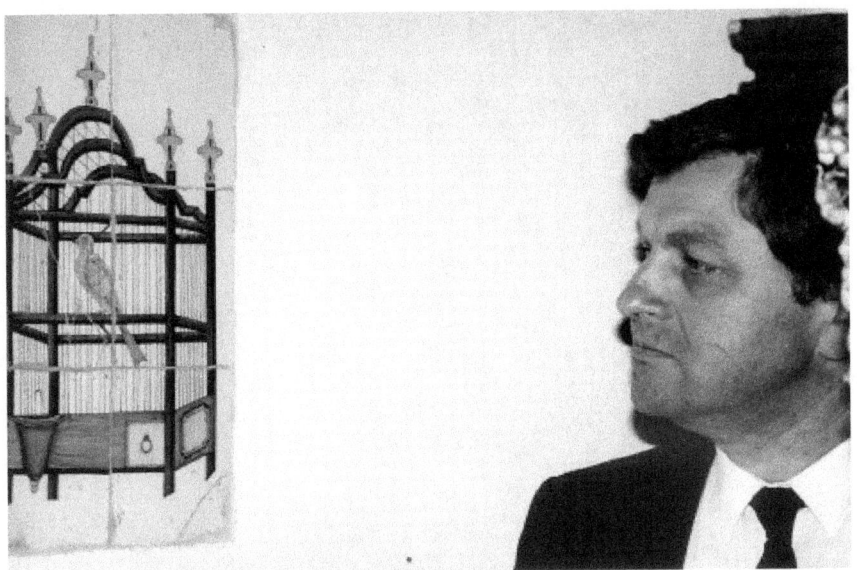

ABOLITION OF ANIMAL Slavery

Paperback 108 pages

E-book

www.youtube.com [1]Peter Holst MD

Preface

─────

I t was not until the mid-twentieth century that life on earth got the reproductive processes under control

The first life forms were found in the Pacific region. 400 million years ago Pan Gaia was surrounded by Pan Ocean. The earth was a huge pancake. Life on Earth has evolved eastward under the influence of gravity, the Earth's rotation and sunrise. Multicellular organisms, fish, marine iguanas and amphibians have emerged from the primordial soup. Dinosaurs, birds, mammals, and monkeys evolved on the land of Pan Gaia. Great apes, homo erectus and homo sapiens originated in Central Africa and Asia.

Homo sapiens has achieved greater manual dexterity in the East African area. The human is the only humanoid who can place the thumb opposite the other fingers and make a precision grip with his hands. The more those hands could do, the more successful their owners were, so the evolutionary pressure created an increasing concentration of nerves and high-precision muscles in the thumb and fingers. The brain grew with it. As a result, people can perform very complex tasks with their hands. Modern man is the first living being to gain control of his reproductive process.

This was followed by control over the reproduction of the herd by applying artificial insemination to the livestock on a large scale

Meat and eggs for consumption in factory farming are still exclusively produced by artificial insemination or using incubators.

Why did we get into a battle against animals?

———

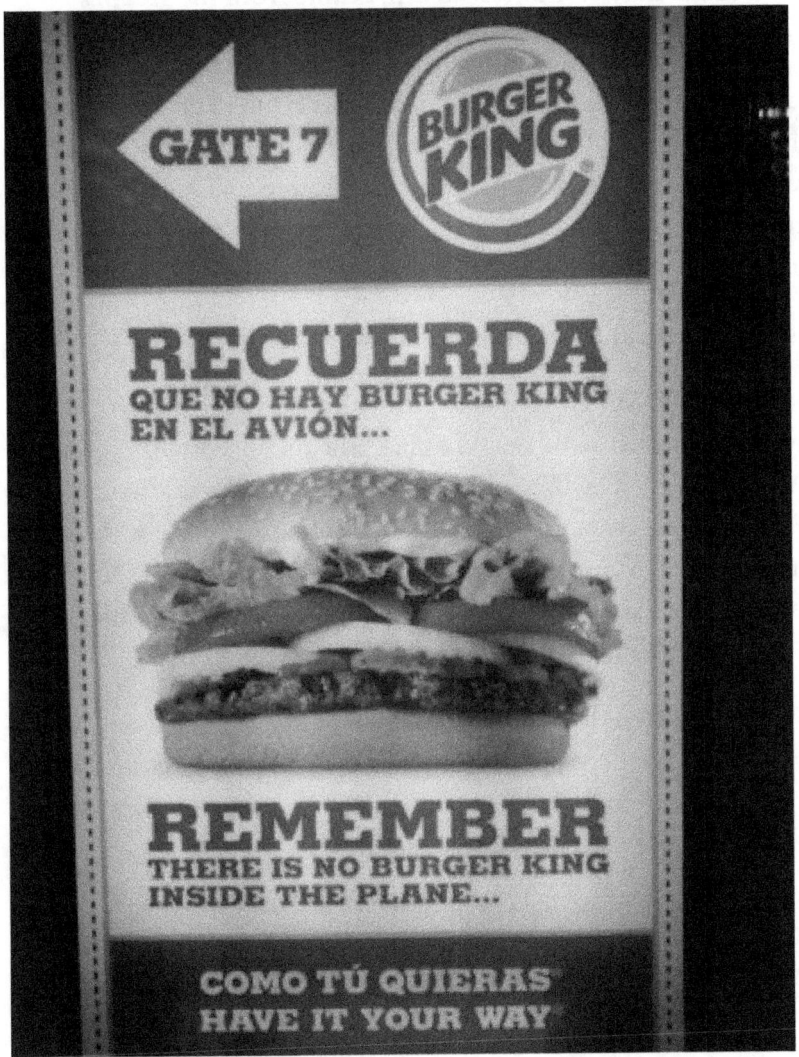

We all know the concept of mass tourism, but what do we know about the mass consumption of cheap burgers and smashers. How did it get so far that we got involved in a fierce battle against the animal army?

Phase 1 of the battle. A bacterial army came from the steppes

The first pandemic was a bacterial pandemic, the bubonic and pneumonic plague in the early Middle Ages (14th century) as a result of the roasting and trading of steppe marmots from Mongolia. The pneumonic plague killed 50% of the European population in the 14th century. The plague bacteria was spread by rats, lice and fleas from the marmot fur.

Phase 2. Viruses and bacteria went to war together

The Spanish flu of 1914 was a virus and bacterial pandemic. The Influenza A (avian) virus caused a flu epidemic in Fort Riley, Kansas, USA. In this fort they bred chickens and pigs for the soldiers. A cook may be infected with the virus. By mutation, the virus was able to cause infection from person to person. Influenza virus (H1N1) was transferred to Europe through millions of deaths via the troop transports of WWII.

The majority of the flu pandemic deaths of 1918-1919 were directly the result of secondary pneumonia caused by common bacteria in the upper respiratory tract. Data from the subsequent pandemics of 1957 and 1968 are consistent with these findings.

Morens DM, Taubenberger JK, Fauci AS. Predominant Role of Bacterial Pneumonia as a Cause of Death in Pandemic Influenza: Implications for Pandemic Influenza Preparedness. J Infect Dis. 2008; 198 (7): 962–70

https://www.ncbi.nlm.nih.gov/pubmed/18710327

Phase 3. Viruses and bats, the flying rats, go to war together

A subsequent pandemic (WHO 1980) was the HIV-1 virus pandemic due to the trade and sale and consumption of chimpanzee bush meat. Since then, HIV / AIDS has resulted in an estimated 65 million infections and 25 million deaths. Especially in Africa. This was followed by the Ebola virus pandemic, also due to the consumption of bush meat and dried bats.

Phase 4. The smallest bacteria go to war from bird cages

After the abolition of slavery, the trade in exotic animals is the new business model. Quartering of bacteria such as Chlamydia pneumoniae in humans. Man is used as a host. Smoking is bad but even more dangerous in the Netherlands, Belgium and England where the highest lung cancer mortality in the world occurs.

Phase 5. RNA viruses and leukemia viruses spread across our food

Humans are used as hosts by these viruses. The billeting of these viruses is responsible for the recent increase in colon and breast cancer. Since the mid-20th century, more and more biofarms have been growing where pigs, cows and rabbits are bred exclusively through artificial insemination.

Phase 6. Corona viruses compete from wet markets

Influenza viruses and coronaviruses are spread mainly from chicken farms, pig fattening and wet markets in SE Asia. Especially the Chinese eat everything that has legs.

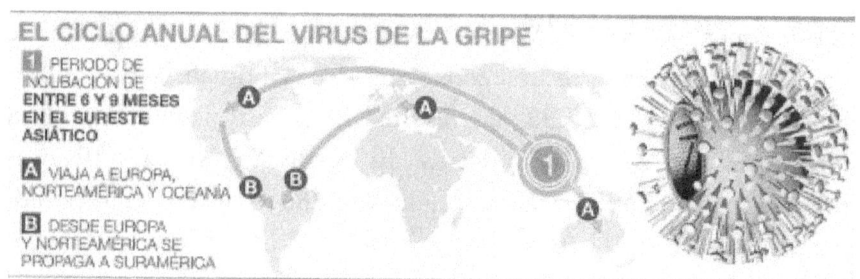

In March 2019 we returned from a cruise in SE Asia, the spice route, and were in Ghuangzhou (Canton) for a few days. On arrival at the airport here our temperature was measured and a woman with a fever was discovered and taken for quarantine. Already a year before the outbreak of COVID-19, temperature measurement and mouth masks were probably already the practice in SE Asia.

Coronaviruses spread like nail bombs in humans and cause many deaths from pneumonia. Bats and rodents spread diseases. Where rats and mice used to transmit diseases, the flying rats (bats) are now the cause of this corona virus pandemic, originating from wildlife in living markets.

Phase 7. David against Goliath

We all know this heroic story from the Bible, it teaches us the lessons we can draw from history. It often seems that the big, the bigger and the biggest are the most challenging, threatening opponents we face on Earth. But David's story teaches us another lesson: the small, the smaller, the smallest creatures can be much stronger than the obvious opponents. Some of them are the viruses and bacteria, they teach us the lessons to be careful what we do, otherwise these little creatures on the brink of life and death will all be the David who will teach us how to behave as humans. And their lessons will and have been hard, as we experience today. If we are stubborn and negligent, we will pay heavily as a gender and as individuals that cause horror and sadness. Is it surprising that we will eventually be beaten by the little ones? The worst of our enemies are in ourselves because of our stubbornness in the struggle for life.

David Attenborough - A Life on Our Planet

Hundreds of studies around the world have confirmed that something is going on. The consequences will be more far-reaching than the pollution of the soil and water in a few countries that are unlucky enough to be caused by explosions at a nuclear power station. The Trump government withdrew from the Paris Climate Agreement. The United States no longer has respect for nature. Half the country is affected by terrible forest fires and they act as if nothing is wrong.

Mankind has come to regard the earth more and more as its property. Including an ever-increasing proportion of wilderness, which has halved worldwide since David Attenborough was a child. We see how the world's population grew and grew, and how almost no one thought about sacrificing his acquired right to a daily piece of meat, resulting in an enormous burden on the environment.

Wild animals are having to make do with less and less living space. Large carnivores - take the lion - are becoming rarer and rarer in the wild, because thanks to man there is less and less habitat for their prey. That law also applies to humans. Our planet cannot cope with our consumption of meat, there is no place for it.

This is the real tragedy of our time: the accelerating decline in the biodiversity of our planet. The greater the biodiversity of our planet, the safer all life on earth, including ourselves, will be. However, biodiversity is plunging under the influence of our current way of life. We lead our pleasant lives in the shadow of a disaster that we ourselves are causing. This catastrophe is caused by the very things that enable us to create an atmosphere of well-being. And it is logical that we will continue to do so until we have a decisive reason to stop doing so, and an appealing alternative. The natural world is in decline. The evidence is convincing it will lead to our destruction. There is another alternative to turn the tide for the better, if we act now.

Part of the solution may well be in the Netherlands, one of the few countries explicitly mentioned in the film. Attenborough explains that it is a densely populated country, but it is still the world's second largest exporter of food. There is no mention of the fact that a large proportion of these exports also involve meat and dairy products. Attenborough shows the efficient way in which vegetables are grown in our country, in greenhouses and under artificial sunlight. That is the future, he thinks.

Our strongest powers, our strongest weapon are our brains, our intellectual capacities. Only use them well, then we can survive! Stop eating factory farm animals. It is high time for humans to adopt different eating habits and stop trading exotic animals and wildlife. Only consume meat from grazing animals or cultured meat from grazing animals. A major advantage of cultured meat is that it offers the possibility to produce meat without having to slaughter animals. In addition, the production of cultured meat is much more efficient, so that more meat can be produced in a laboratory in a shorter time than with regular livestock farming. About ten thousand kilos of meat can be made with the stem cells of one gram of muscle tissue. In theory this means that the stem cells of one hundred and fifty cows can be used to feed the whole world. Mosa Meat and Nutreco want to enter the market with cultured meat in 2022.

They make beef from the muscle cells of an animal, such as a cow. The cells proliferate until trillions of cells from a small sample. This growth takes place in a bioreactor, which looks similar to the bioreactors that beer and yoghurt are fermented in. From one sample from a cow, they can produce 800 million strands of muscle tissue (enough to make 80.000 quarter pounders).

Index

Lessons from the past

Civet cats

The SARS epidemic, between November 2002 and July 2003, resulted in about 8,000 infections. Nearly eight hundred people died. Severe Acute Respiratory Syndrome spread over more than thirty countries, including Europe. Outside of China, Hong Kong, Canada, Taiwan and Singapore were hardest hit. In China, almost all provinces were affected. The Netherlands remained free from SARS. Guangdong Province (Canton) was the heart of this pandemic in 2002. Breeding, trading and eating of civets has been banned in Guangdong since January 2004. The Guangdong government has been checking for years whether pet markets or restaurants have civets, in cages or in the freezer. However, recent inspections have shown that civet cats are still traded by restaurants in the Guandong Province and also Hubei Province (Wuhan), as revealed in December 2019.

Coronaviruses and pneumonia

The SARS virus that emerged in China in 2003 and spread through the civet, the MERS virus came from dromedaries and has been active since 2012, and the SARS coronavirus II that now caused a pandemic as COVID 19 are three new viruses of this century that have dangerous pneumonia and give death.

Intensive goat breeding and Q fever pneumonia

Manure and straw from the goats are distributed by farmers as fertilization over the land. Infected pregnant milk goats spread spores of the bacteria, after giving birth, with the afterbirth and amniotic fluid in the straw. As a result, the Coxiella-burnetii bacterium and spores spread through the air, infecting the local population in North Brabant, even after inhaling 100 germs.

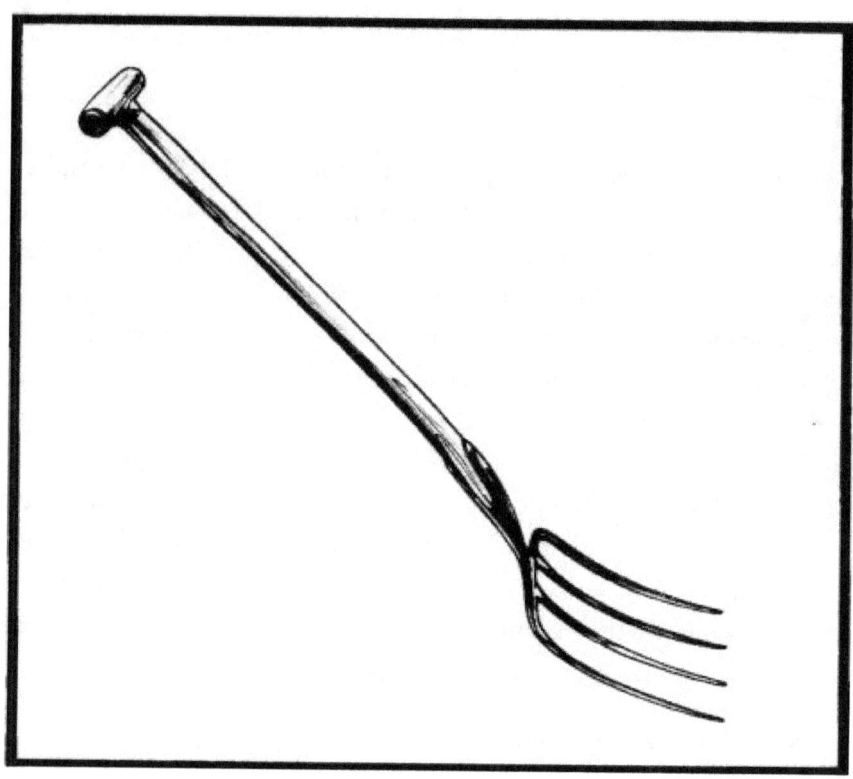

Grip, multi-toothed manure fork

Lung cancer in The Netherlands, Belgium and UK

Country	Cigarette packs of 20 per year in 1970	Lung cancer mortality 1984 (CBS NL) 2010 (EUROSTAT)	
Italy	84	77	73
Norway	88	43	71
France	92	65	87
Finland	93	87	73
Netherlands	**108**	**117**	**108**
Belgium	**119**	**119**	**115**
West Germany	125	73	West & East Germany 79
Japan	*141*	*43*	
United Kingdom	**153**	**100**	**82**
USA	*184*	*84*	

Age standardized lung cancer mortality (ICD 162 per 100,000 men per year) in ten different countries in 1984, 2007 and 2010 in relation to per adult consumption of manufactured / hand-rolled cigarettes in 1970.

- **In Japan and the USA has always been a lot more smoking and mortality rates of lung cancer were lower.**

In 2012, cancer was the cause of 31% of all deaths in the Netherlands (Eurostat). Today about half of all men and one third of all women develop cancer and about 20% of all deaths are due to cancer. This is an impressive increase and seems to show that the increase in cancer is a recent biological event.

- **More lung cancer in The Netherlands, Belgium and the United Kingdom. These three countries have the largest share in the international trade and import of tropical birds via Amsterdam Schiphol, Brussels Zaventem and London Heathrow respectively.**

In 2019, 14,000 people in the Netherlands developed lung cancer

Only 3,000 of these will be alive in 2024 (19% survival rate after five years). Lung cancer is not contagious but demands a lot from health care year after year. Every day 128 people die of cancer in the Netherlands. Cancer has been the leading cause of death in our country since the beginning of the 21st century. After colon cancer, the chance of being alive after five years is about 60%. For breast cancer, the chance of being alive after five years is about 85%, much more favorable than for lung cancer.

Netherlands, Belgium and the United Kingdom have the highest lung cancer mortality of any country in Europe. Besides smoking, the hobby and breeding of tropical birds are the reason for this excess mortality.

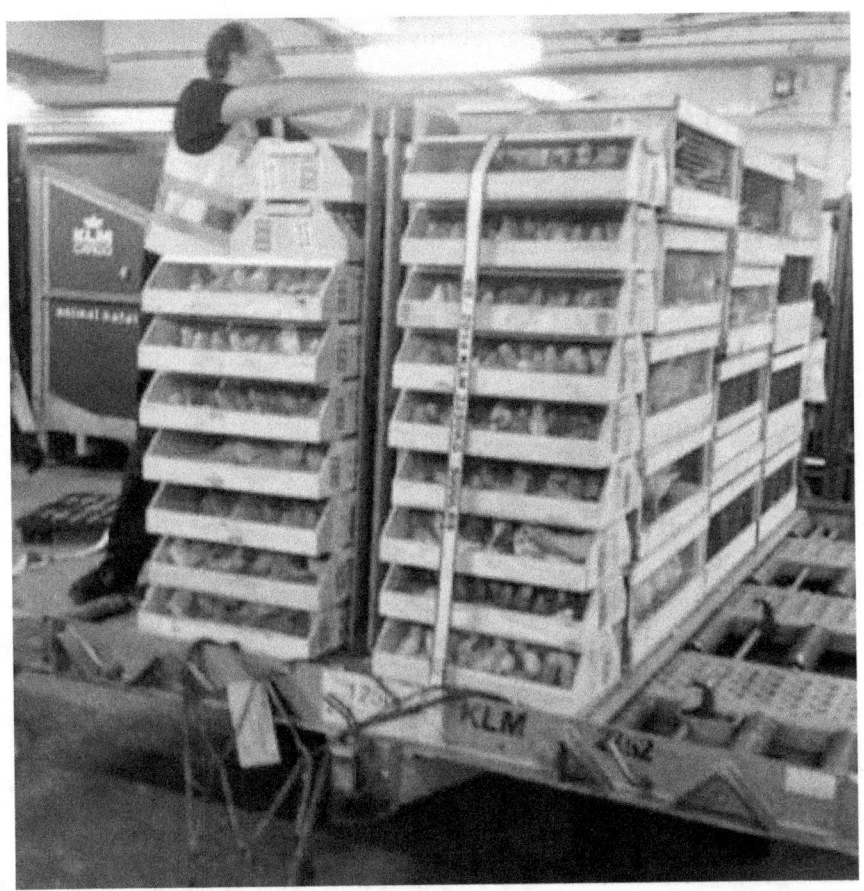

Bird exhibitions and bird breeders caused an explosive growth of this popular hobby

Since the slave trade and slavery were abolished 150 years ago, international trade in tropical companion animals, international human trafficking, the arms industry and drug trafficking became the most profitable forms of trade. Worldwide, an estimated 40,000 primates, 4 million exotic birds, 640,000 reptiles and 350 million tropical fish are traded live each year. The trade in exotics is estimated at an $ 6 billion industry. Bird exhibitions and bird breeders caused an explosive growth of this popular hobby

Keeping and breeding tropical birds is a hobby of young families. The ratio of breeders to the total number of bird keepers is about 1: 6. The level of organization of the large bird breeders in the Netherlands is high due to participation in the breeding competitions. Public shows, which were held several times a year, made the hobby increasingly popular in the twentieth century. When pigeons are kept together with tropical birds, Chlamydia infections are more common.

In the Netherlands were 7.5 million birds in households in 1984. The American Veterinary Medicine Association (AVMA) counted 11-16 million companion birds and exotic birds in the United States in 2007. In France, 6 million companion birds were owned by households in 2010. In Belgium every bred bird must be provided with a ring with a number to which the owner can identify the breeder. In 2011 the Association Ornithologique de Belgique (AOB) registered 249 ornithological associations. Exotic birds such as larger parrots, macaw or cockatoo are traded legally or illegally from Asia or South America. These birds are still high on the list of popular pets and are also richly represented in zoos and parks.

Tropical birds were late in history brought to the Old World. Increasingly larger numbers were taken as trophies bysailors, after the colonization of South America and the Caribbean. Only with the increase of shipping traffic and air cargo, tropical birds could easily be imported and traded in Europe. The largest epidemic of psittacosis occurred in 1929-1930 after the import of infected parrots from Argentina to Europe. Hundreds of people became seriously ill and 20% died after an acute fulminant disease. Initially, in many countries strict import restrictions were set. Not much later parrots were again massively imported. Bird shows and bird breeders produced an explosive growth of this popular pastime. The housing of tropical birds in Western Europe has led to the adaptation of the psittacosis "virus", first in the flocks of the pigeon breeders who often kept also tropical birds. With many tropical bird breeders the 'psittacosis virus' adapted and the disease that occurred in humans was less violent.

The Chlamydia pneumoniae has adapted in Western Europe and the epidemic of bird flu (ornithosis) and Chlamydia pneumonia were the result of this. Chlamydia pneumonia is adjusted so that this microorganism now also passes from human to human through the airways and is now so prevalent in society that 98% have been infected. Repeated infections with Chlamydiae, primarily occurring with bird breeders and bird keepers cause chronic respiratory diseases and cause lung cancer in humans.

On the accompanying map there is more particulate matter in the air in the red places. In North Brabant this is caused by the many pig stables, the goat breeders, the many bird breeders and the mink farms.

Particulate matter 2.5 and Covid-19 cases

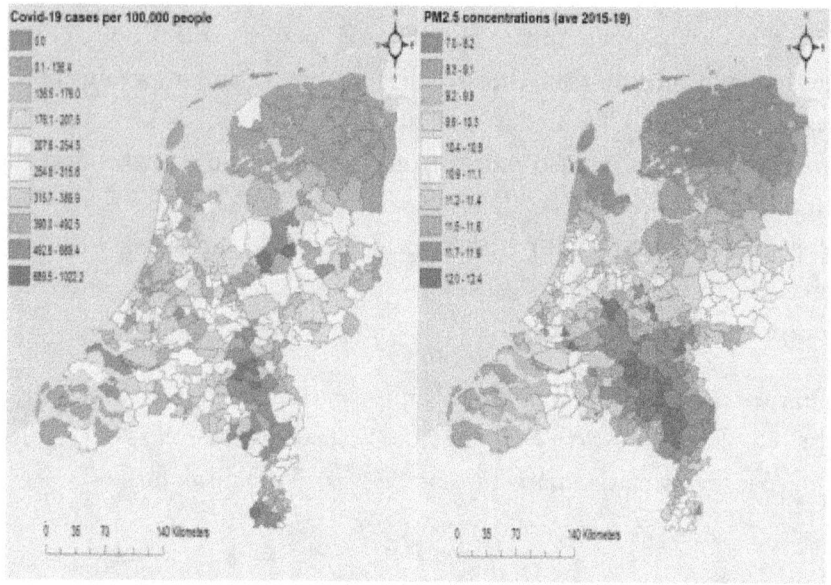

In late February and early March each year carnival celebrations attract thousands of people to street parties and parades – 2020 was no exception, so does that explain the rapid spread of COVID-19 in North Brabant? While it's likely that the carnival celebrations played a role, the pattern of cases across these regions suggest other factors may be at least as important.

The south-eastern provinces of North Brabant and Limburg house over 63% of the country's 12 million pigs and 42% of its 101 million chickens. Intensive livestock production produces large amounts of ammonia. These particles often form a significant proportion of fine particulate in air pollution. Concentrations are at highest in air samples from the south-east of the Netherlands.

Why North Brabant?

It is dangerous to smoke, but more dangerous in Belgium, the Netherlands and United Kingdom. Especially in the east of North Brabant in the surrounding of Tilburg it is most dangerous to smoke. Is this due to the carnival or is there more going on?

O rganised bird breeders as at 1-1-1984 per province

North Brabant (male population 1.054.281) 23.009

South Holland (1.539.994) 15.612

Gelderland (859.840) 14.638

Limburg (540.669) 12.426

Overijssel (519.800) 10.096

North Holland (1.123.305) 8.973

Utrecht (454.452) 6.966

Friesland (269.902) 5.223

Zeeland (176.736) 5.046

Groningen (278.747) 4.952

Drenthe (213.472) 3.726

Netherlands (male population 7.067.198) 110.667

Most of the bird clubs and organized birdkeepers are traditionally found in North Brabant, above all in Tilburg. There are regional differences in the Netherlands in male lung cancer mortality that cannot be explained by differences in the age distribution of the population. Unfortunately, regional information about smoking habits is not available. The rural province of North Brabant had, in 1984, the highest age-standardized lung cancer mortality. This province contains three towns among the eight largest municipalities with the highest lung cancer mortality in the Netherlands. Tilburg and Maastricht had the highest standardized lung cancer mortality among the eight largest municipalities for the years 1969-1978 (CBS 1980). Tilburg also had the highest mortality in 1984. Most of the bird clubs and most of the organized birdkeepers are traditionally found in North Brabant. The number of organized bird breeders of the Netherlands society of bird lovers grew dramatically from 1.400 in the year 1940 to 45.800 in 1984.

It is dangerous to smoke, but more dangerous to smoke in Tilburg

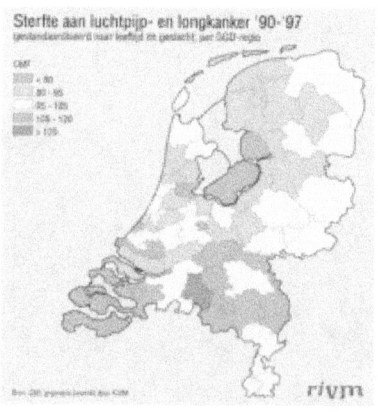

- Since 1969, the province of North Brabant had the highest age-standardised lung cancer mortality.

- Most of the bird clubs and organised birdkeepers are traditionally found in this province, above all in Tilburg

- Also from 1990 until 1997 North Brabant had the highest lung cancer mortality in the Netherlands and again Tilburg

LUNG CANCER MORTALITY (per 100000 men per year) in different Dutch provinces and large municipalities

Province	Municipality	1969 -1978	1984
North Brabant		91	114
	Tilburg	117	131
	Eindhoven	98	121
	Breda	98	117
Utrecht		89	109
Limburg		93	104
	Maastricht	103	92
Overijssel		75	104
North-Holland		95	104
	Haarlem	11	114
	Amsterdam	100	104
South-Holland		92	103
	Rotterdam	102	123
	Leiden	99	102
Gelderland		77	102
Groningen		67	90
Friesland		62	89
Drenthe		60	88
Zeeland		60	86

From 1990 until 1997 North Brabant had again the highest lung cancer mortality in the Netherlands and again Tilburg.

The incidence of lung cancer was quite low in the Netherlands until 1950. In 1950, 1.179 men and 167 women died from this disease. By 1983, the numbers had increased to 7.104 men and 800 women. Standardized for age, the mortality per 100.000 men increased from 27 to 120 between 1950 and 1988 and per 100.000 women from 3.3 to 10.6 during this period.

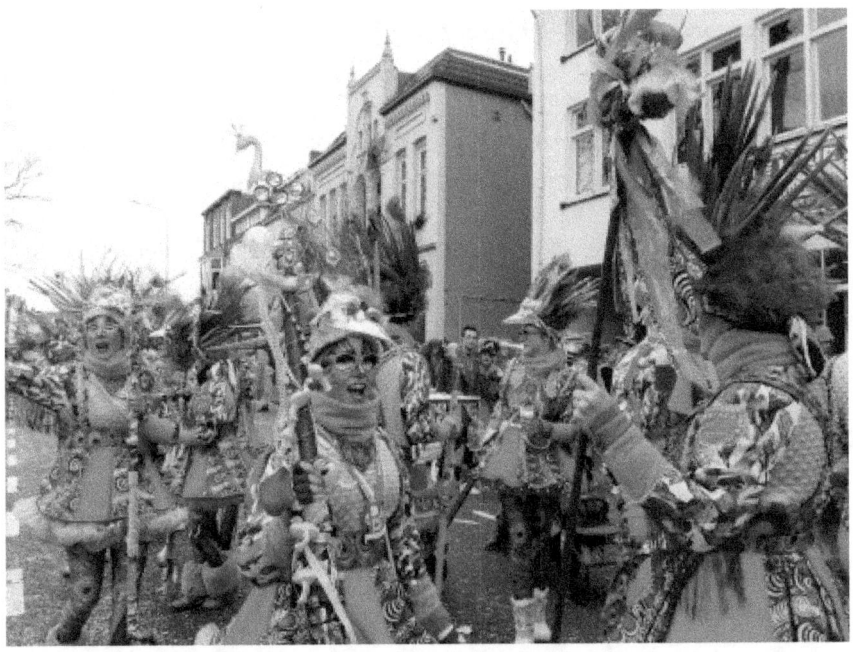

Due to the rural character (which correlates with Carnival traditions) there are many pig stables and goat farmers at the locations of the Carnival. So distribution does not even have to be via carnival gatherings. Most large floats are made and parked precisely IN the stables of farms, and the makers of them frolic everywhere through the mud and straw the day before, shake the farmer's hand and eat another sandwich there. Then embrace each other during parades and also the public along the way.

Why were most Covid-19 infections in North Brabant?

It seems like a big mystery: the corona outbreak in North Brabant. The province is increasingly developing into a source of fire for the virus in the Netherlands. Why most people got infected here?

A year ago, we were at a wedding party near Eindhoven. I walked outside with the idea to enjoy a clear evening. The sky was so polluted with dust that no stars were visible, and there was a pungent smell of neighboring pig fattening farms. How is the indoor air in the houses of the many pigeon fanciers, goat breeders, pig farmers and mink farmers. In a bad indoor climate, the flu will spread quickly to family members and friends. How is the indoor climate in the many pig slaughterhouses where temperature fluctuates, needs to be worked quickly in a noisy environment and often shout at each other. In Germany and the United States also many workers in slaughterhouses and meatpacking industries have proven to be infected with Covid-19 from March to June 2020.

During the carnival, the corona virus entered a melting pot of visitors. The risk of contamination is particularly high within banquet halls and bars.

Why could Covid-19 get this far in China?

The African Swine Fever pandemic started in 2007 when it entered Georgia (Caucasus region of Eurasia), most probably by the feeding of local pigs with ASF-contaminated swill, which included pork remains unloaded from a ship arriving from west Africa. Since then, it has spread, eventually infecting domestic pigs and wild boar, throughout vast parts of Eurasia. Its most recent further spread involved India. The African swine fever (ASF) pandemic will be even worse this year [2020] than in 2019, say experts, warning that the spread of the highly contagious virus, which is fatal to pigs, is unrelenting.

With world attention on the human viral pandemic of COVID-19, concern is growing that countries are not focusing enough on halting the spread of ASF through better biosecurity practices, cooperation on intensive vaccine development, or transparency regarding outbreaks.

"The ASF virus is a much 'stronger' virus than Covid-19, in that it can survive in the environment or processed meat for weeks and months. ASF kills almost 100% of the animals it infects, and despite being in circulation for nearly 100 years, there is still no vaccine. African swine fever outbreaks have occurred in several provinces of China since August 2018. At the end of 2018, the total number of culled animals was 650,000. The pig herd of China, by far the largest in the world, was estimated at 360 million animals at the time. The number of pigs was half, a year earlier by the end of 2019, as an epidemic of African swine fever spread among the largest pork producer in the world. About 200 million pigs were culled or died as a result of the disease, while pork production fell by 40%. Production may take more than 5 years to

31

recover to previous levels before the deadly outbreaks, due to a lack of solutions to prevent the disease and a lack of capital to form new stocks.

Currently, focal locations of the virus are primarily in China, Vietnam, the Philippines, and a wide swath of Eastern Europe. The disease has now spread to northern India for the 1st time as well as to Papua New Guinea. Recent outbreaks among wild boar populations in Belgium, now under control, have also heightened monitoring in Western Europe.

There are also concerns that China is underreporting the data for 2020. "We see ASF every week here," Wayne Johnson, veterinarian at farm services company Enable Agricultural Technology Consulting, who is based in Beijing. "Provinces are told not to report. China does not report anything that would give [an] accurate account." China has now gone from culling to controlling and living with it. "The benefit that the ASF epidemic has had for the financial performance of the mega pig producers in China adds another interesting dimension to the story. They have actually learned to 'live' with the disease in the country and benefit enormously from the high pork price." Profits continue to skyrocket at top Chinese pork producers such as WH Group, Wens, and Muyuan. Fears are growing among pig producers in the US and Europe that it is only a matter of time before the disease reaches their pig herds from continuing outbreaks in China, Southeast Asia, and Eastern Europe. It's just whether that somebody would put [contaminated meat] in a bin or chuck something over a hedge that the pigs got access to.

At the end of 2019, there was a first outbreak of a new coronavirus in Wuhan, which has been the source of this virus ever since. The Corona SARS 2 virus has jumped from animal to man in a market in the Chinese metropolis of Wuhan. On the Wuhan live animal market, exotic animals such as snakes, turtles, bats, foxes and porcupines are sold for consumption. Even civets, a feline creature, are still bred intensively and were on an extensive price list of the animal trading companies on the market in Wuhan. The virus is housed and spread by bats, which are cooked alive for soup in China and elsewhere in the world. It is very unfortunate that the Year of the Rat 2020 in China starts with a new coronavirus epidemic, caused by bats, also known as the flying rats. After the 2013 SARS epidemic, which spread from Hong Kong, Chinese virologists previously warned that bat-borne coronaviruses would reappear to cause the next outbreak of the disease. China is a hot spot. Bats are an incredibly diverse group that makes up a quarter of all mammals, rodents count 50 percent, and we humans are in the remaining 25% of mammals. Bats live on every continent, close to people and farms. Slaughtered animals are fattened as quickly as possible to maximize food production. The bats' ability to fly provides them with a wide habitat. Their droppings can spread disease. Bats are host to a higher proportion of zoonoses than all other mammals. Their ability to coexist with viruses that can spill over to other mammals, in particular humans, can have devastating consequences when we eat them, trade them in livestock markets, and invade their territory. People in many parts of the world eat bats and sell them in live animal markets.

- Stopping the sale of wildlife in markets is essential to curtail future outbreaks of diseases that spill over from animals to humans.
- **The decision, taken by the Chinese National People's Congress on February 24, 2020, that illegal consumption and trade in wild animals will be "severely punished", as well as hunting, trade or transportation of wild animals for consumption is more necessary than ever.**

The SARS epidemic, between November 2002 and July 2003, resulted in about 8,000 infections. Nearly eight hundred people died. Severe

Acute Respiratory Syndrome spread over more than thirty countries, including Europe. Outside of China, Hong Kong, Canada, Taiwan and Singapore were hardest hit. In China, almost all provinces were affected. The Netherlands remained free from SARS. Guangdong Province (Canton) was the heart of this pandemic in 2002. Breeding, trading and eating of civets has been banned in Guangdong since January 2004. The Guangdong government has been checking for years whether pet markets or restaurants have civets, in cages or in the freezer. However, recent inspections have shown that civet cats are still traded by restaurants in the Guandong Province and also Hubei Province (Wuhan), as revealed in December 2019.

Coronaviruses and pneumonia

The SARS virus that emerged in China in 2003 and spread through the civet, the MERS virus came from dromedaries and has been active since 2012, and the SARS coronavirus II that now caused a pandemic as COVID 19 are three new viruses of this century that have dangerous pneumonia and give death.

Results in treatment of Covid-19 pneumonia

The coronavirus is a miniscule little nail bomb that is able to invade living body cells and take advantage of host cell protein synthesis and to produce offspring allowing hundreds of new virus particles to exit the host cell and spread throughout the body, resulting in a mortally ill patient. Several treating physicians have reported success in the treatment of patients with fever and COVID-19 pneumonia with Azithromycin. Azithromycin, a macrolide antibiotic, erythromycin and also doxycycline prevent viruses from multiplying by interfering with their protein synthesis in the host cell. It binds to the ribosomes in the host cell, inhibiting the transport of RNA and protein synthesis from viruses, preventing multiplication and spread in the body. The majority of deaths in the 1918–1919 influenza pandemic likely resulted directly from secondary bacterial pneumonia caused by common upper respiratory-tract bacteria. Data from the subsequent 1957 and 1968 pandemics are consistent with these findings. Antibiotics have also proven to favorably influence the course of the disease in pneumonia during these influenza epidemics. In the time of the 1918-1919 pandemic there was no antibiotic. Alexander Fleming discovered penicillin only in 1928.

Morens DM, Taubenberger JK, Fauci AS. Predominant Role of Bacterial Pneumonia as a Cause of Death in Pandemic Influenza: Implications for Pandemic Influenza Preparedness. J Infect Dis. 2008 Oct 1;198(7): 962–70

https://www.ncbi.nlm.nih.gov/pubmed/18710327

Patients with COVID-19 have been reported to be similarly at risk of secondary bacterial pneumonia, either as a consequence of damage inflicted by the novel coronavirus itself or invasive procedures such as intubation/mechanical ventilation to manage respiratory failure. Long-term immobilization in intensive care has also led to thrombosis and embolization.

Not only giving paracetamol with this rapidly progressing respiratory tract infection but giving an adequate antibiotic such as azithromycin or doxycycline immediately with a fever can prevent worse.

The impact of air pollution on health.

In January 2013, China suffered large-scale haze weather four times, affecting 30 cities in all. The average number of haze weather days in many regions was higher than the same period in every year since 1961. Hong Kong has only four weeks a year without smog because of the air pollution that comes over from the south of China. **PM2.5, which is defined as fine particulate matter with an aerodynamic diameter of 2.5 micrometers or less, is the main health hazard of smog.** Smog can carry large amounts of poisonous and harmful substances and penetrate deep into the lungs and blood circulation through the respiratory tract, thereby affecting human health. The Global Burden of Disease Study 2010 ranked particulate matter as the 8th highest cause of death worldwide, when considering estimated deaths attributable to the independent effects of 67 risk factors. In China, this ranking could be as high as 4th, accounting for approximately 1.2 million premature deaths in 2010.

The health effects of haze weather studies mainly focus on PM2.5 particles. Environmental epidemiology research in recent decades has proved that short or long-term exposure to ambient PM2.5 particulate matter was associated with increased mortality and morbidity, reduction in life expectancy and additional respiratory and cardiovascular diseases. PM2.5 could penetrate deeply into the lungs through the respiratory tract due to its small size and irritate and corrode the alveolar wall. The resulting impaired lung function would show as coughs, wheezes, respiratory disorders and other symptoms, and increase the risks of bronchial asthma, chronic obstructive pulmonary disease (COPD), emphysema and other respiratory diseases.

Indoor Air Pollution

Significantly increased dust levels are measured in households where birds are kept. Particulate matter with a diameter of 2.5 micron or less is the most important health risk of (indoor) air pollution. The number of particles of about 2 microns is increased in bird-keeping households. Bird keepers, and especially bird breeders, have an increased risk of infection with local damage to the tissue and allergic reactions in the lung tissue. Due to excessive mucus production, there is more drainage of alveoli in smokers than in non-smokers. As a result, the dust container and antigen load is shifted from the alveoli to the smaller air tubes in the bird keeper who smokes. The antigens reach the smallest alveoli in smaller quantities and the immune responses and inflammation occur more strongly in smaller bronchi.

- **The smaller bronchi are the preferred location of lung cancer**

Both smoking and keeping birds are ultimately responsible for the poor functioning of the "lung cleaning service" and a shortage of immune proteins. The result is less protection of the lung mucosal cells against continual allergen and fine material that precipitates on the thin mucus layer of the smaller air tubes and subsequently lung cancer. It is therefore possible to see why most lung tumors develop in the smaller air tubes, at some distance from the finest alveoli, where gases and dust particles circulate at first instance. Both smoking and keeping birds at home increases the dust content of the air in the house.

- **Dust particles from bird cages and tobacco smoke are potentially more harmful than the particles that occur in**

outside air (eg pollen grains, ash, soot particles and sand grains)

- There is every reason to pay particular attention to the bird breeders among the smokers.

Felderhof-Hoytema (1987) followed 699 school children aged 4 to 16 in The Hague. Of these children, 39.6% had birds at home. In children with one or more cage birds at home, 50.9% had symptoms of Chronic Non-Specific Lung Disease compared to 19% in children without cage birds at home. Converted, this means that 50% of the more serious forms of CNSLD, are related to the presence of cage birds at home.

- It is more obvious to measure particulate matter levels in households with birds than in classrooms.

Chlamydia pneumoniae and lung cancer

———

L ong-term studies using cigarette smoking machines, in hamsters, dogs and monkeys, did not show a statistically significant increase in malignant tumors in the airways, although very long exposures and high doses of smoke were used (Coggins CR 2001). These inhalation studies were performed without additional respiratory infection of the test animals. The tobacco industry has long cited the studies as evidence of no increase in lung cancer from smoking.

An animal model for lung cancer was developed by repeated injection of Chlamydia pneumonia into rat airways, with or without the most carcinogenic component of the cigarette benzo (a) pyrene (Chu DJ 2012). With the combination of benzo (a) pyrene and the bacteria of tropical bird flu in the spray, 44% of the laboratory rats developed lung cancer. The combined factors of smoking and chronic Cp infection have effects on each other and lead to a greatly increased risk of lung cancer.

Chu DJ, Guo SG, Pan CF, Wang J, Du Y, Lu XF, Yu ZY (2012) An experimental model for induction of lung cancer in rats by Chlamydia pneumoniae.

Asian Pac J Cancer Prev. 2012; 13 (6): 2819-22 https://www.ncbi.nlm.nih.gov/pubmed/22938465

Favorable results of combined therapy of azithromycin with the chemotherapy on non-small cell lung cancer patients

Although new chemotherapeutic drugs have been applied constantly, their efficacy for non-small cell lung cancer (NSCLC) is still not satisfactory. In recent years, epidemiological investigations have shown that lung cancer may be induced by chronic Chlamydia pneumonia (Cpn) infection. This study (Chu DJ 2014) of azithromycin, commonly used for the treatment of Cp infections, combined with the chemotherapeutics paclitaxe and cisplatin on stage III-IV NSCLC patients achieved favorable results in terms of side effects and overall survival.

How are infections related to lung cancer?

Smallest bacteria as Chlamydiae and retroviruses are related to the development of lung cancer. Half of the biomass on earth exists of monomers. Unicellular organisms such as bacteria, yeast cells, amoebae and viruses divide themselves interminable. Tumor cell lines share this property. Multi-cellular organisms have this property only in their stem cells and germ cells. All other cells die after about 50 cell divisions. Of the unicellular organisms, smallest spore forming bacteria as Chlamydiae and viruses are obligate cell parasites. They are the most successful and efficient in reproduction of their genome (Clark 1996). That detracts nothing from the fact that they first need to infect a living cell. When Chlamydiae enter bronchus epithelial cells they remain latent and persistent. When they integrate in the genome of the basal epithelial cell they could lead to the development of a tumour cell. After about 30 tumour cell divisions there is a discernible tumour. These processes take at least 10-15 years.

Chlamydial infection of the human respiratory tract was first described over 100 years ago, when outbreaks of psittacosis were linked to from Argentina in Western Europe imported pet birds. The causative agent was identified subsequently as Chlamydia psittaci. It was once thought that birds imported from abroad, often illegally, were a principal source, but many domestic breeder flocks of pet birds now have become infected. Because of the popularisation of bird keeping during the past century people introduced more and more pet birds and their accompanying obligate cell parasites in their own home environment. Young couples keep sometimes birds in their bedroom. Not seldom a cage bird is placed in a child's room. Most infections in humans are due to exposure to psittacine birds and pigeons; however, outbreaks resulting in severe disease and even death do occur in abattoir workers following processing of infected flocks. Data also indicate that vertical transmission may occur. Persistently infected carrier birds are known to be a source of Chlamydiae in the pet industry. Infections with Chlamydia psittaci from human to human do occur. Chlamydia pneumoniae (strain TWAR) has also been recognised recently as an important cause of human respiratory tract infection. Antibodies to the TWAR strains have so far been detected only in humans but not in birds or domestic or pet animals suggesting humans as the sole host for these organisms. It seems that Chlamydiae have a great adaptability to their hosts.

Chlamydiae pneumoniae were found to be serologically associated with lung cancer (Laurila 1997; Koyi 1999; Jackson 2000)

Laurila et al. found chronic Chlamydia pneumoniae infection in 52% of lung cancer patients (n=230) and in 45% of controls. The incidence was especially increased in men younger than 60 years (OR 2.9; 95% C.I. 1.5-5.4) but not in the older age group (OR 0.9; 95% C.I. 0.5-1.6). Koyi et al. found Chlamydia pneumoniae significant more often in patients with lung cancer (n=117) than in control groups. Jackson et al. found Chlamydia pneumoniae IgA antibody titre 216 independently associated with risk of lung cancer (143 cases) among subjects < 60 years of age (OR 2.67; 95% C.I. 1.21-5.89) but not among older subjects (OR 0.69; 95% C.I. 0.34-1.43).

14.000 in Netherlands developed lung cancer in 2019

Only 3.000 of these people will be alive in 2024 (19% survival rate after five years). Lung cancer is not contagious but demands a lot from health care year after year. Every day 128 people die of cancer in the Netherlands. Cancer has been the leading cause of death in our country since the beginning of the 21st century. After colon cancer, the chance of being alive after five years is about 60%. For breast cancer, the chance of being alive after five years is about 85%, much more favorable than for lung cancer.

Netherlands, Belgium and the United Kingdom have the highest lung cancer mortality of any country in Europe. Besides smoking, the hobby and breeding of tropical birds are the reason for this excess mortality.

Results for treatment of persistent cell infections with Chlamydia

Malignant lymphomas were treated with tetracycline (doxycycline) and their disappearance was accompanied by the eradication of the Chlamydia pneumonia bacteria detected in the cells (Ferreri AJ 2005). This cell infection can be controlled and prevented. Penicillin kills bacteria by preventing the bacteria from rebuilding their cell wall after division. The Chlamydia bacterium has no cell wall and, like viruses, is completely dependent on mucous membrane cells in the airways. By entering a body cell, the bacteria come to life. Then it will copy itself. In the end, hundreds of new bacteria leave the cell and spread further into the airways and body.

Healing of malignant lymphoma with doxycycline

Chlamydia psittaci (Cp), the bacterium of psittacose has often been shown in malignant lymphomas. The bacterium has been shown in the tumor tissue, taken out and cell cultures are made. By treatment with doxycycline (tetracycline) malignant lymphomas are cured (Ferreri AJ). Treatment with doxycycline (twice daily 100 mg) for six months disappeared the malignant lymphomas in 64% of patients. Tetracycline and macrolide (erythromycin) antibiotics have a remarkable therapeutic effect on Cp infection. Cp infection is thus controllable. Chlamydiae have no cell wall and, like viruses, are completely dependent on their host cells. Once in the host cell, Chlamydiae is not sensitive to penicillin. Tetracycline enters cells in the contaminated body cells by diffusion along membrane pores. Once in the cell, tetracyclines and doxycycline inhibit internal cell metabolism, DNA and protein synthesis, whereby Chlamydia cell parasites cannot create new proteins for growth and proliferation.

Ferreri AJ, Ponzoni M, Guidoboni M et al. (2006) Bacteria-eradicating therapy with doxycycline in ocular adnexal MALT lymphoma: a multicenter prospective trial. J Natl Cancer Inst 98:1375– 1382.

https://www.ncbi.nlm.nih.gov/pubmed/15968003

Ferreri AJ, Govi S, Pasini E et al. (2012) Chlamydophila Psittaci Eradication with Doxycycline as first-line targeted therapy for Ocular Adnexae Lymphoma: Final Results of an International Phase II Trial. J Clin Oncol 3

https://www.ncbi.nlm.nih.gov/pubmed/22802315

How could meat production increase so fast in the West?

T*he increase in meat products and dairy production in the West could only be achieved with artificial insemination of mammals and the animals unilaterally fattening with soy flour, corn and fish meal.*

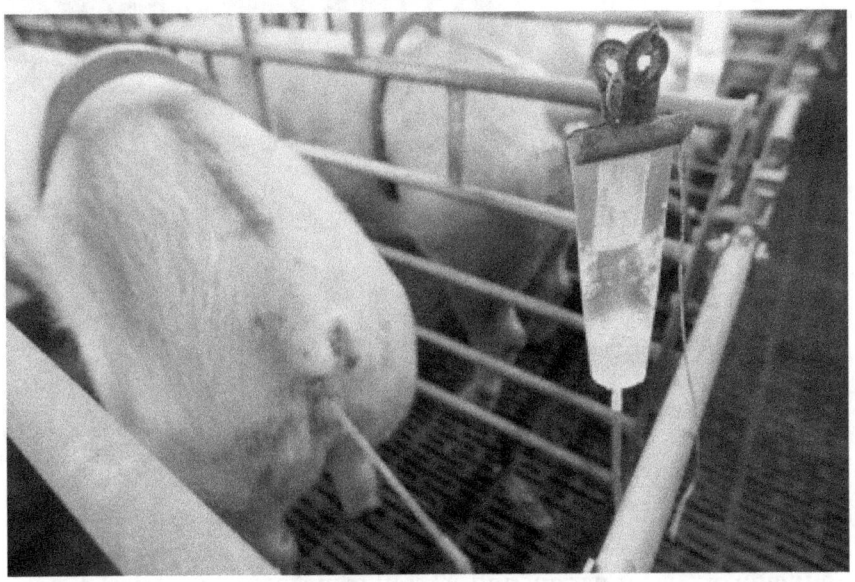

Artificial insemination of pigs in a factory farm

The unbridled breeding of animals, through artificial insemination of cattle and with incubators for poultry, has a devastating effect on our health, nature and the climate. Fast food, unnatural food and meat consumption lead to obesity, vitamin deficiencies, chronic diseases and premature death. Cancer is now the main cause of premature death.

WHAT ARE THE RISKS of higher meat production?

An increased mortality of brain tumors has been observed in veterinary surgeons (Blair A). Veterinarians and Artificial Insemination assistants do a lot of internal research on cows. Transmission via the uterus and the birth canal during labor, of bovine leukemia virus (BLV) plays a crucial role in the spread and persistence of BLV infection in cattle.

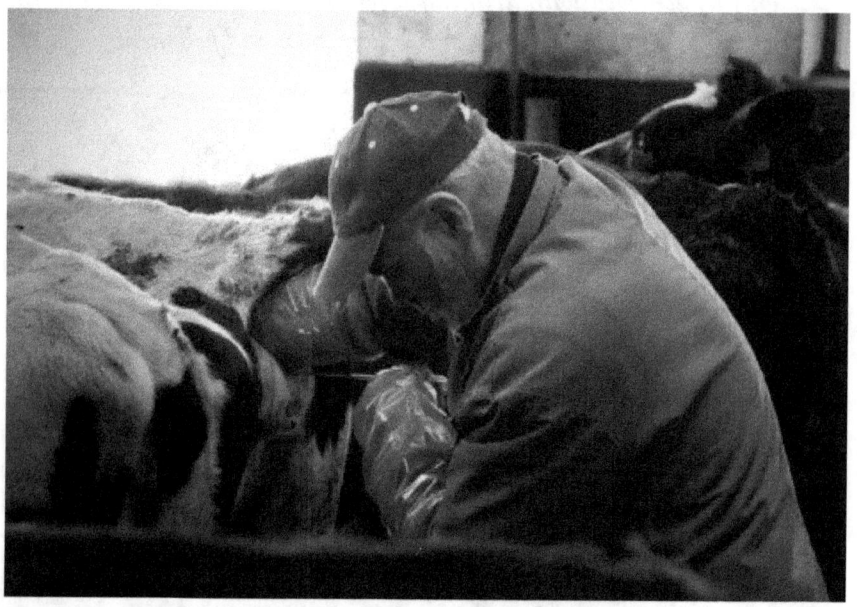

In their work, veterinarians and AI staff come into contact with bovine leukemia virus (BLV), a carcinogenic virus. Bovine leukemia is an economically important infection of dairy cattle worldwide. The presence of infections in Canadian dairy herds is high and is still increasing. Seventy percent of the herds were identified as BLV positive (one or more positive animals).

Nekouei O, VanLeeuwen J, Sanchez J, Kelton D, Tiwari A, Keefe G Herd-level risk factors for infection with bovine leukemia virus in Canadian dairy herds. Prev Vet Med. 2015; 119 (3-4)

The deaths of 5,016 veterinarians were examined and compared with those of the general American population. The mortality rates were significantly increased from malignant lymphomas and leukemia, colon, brain and skin. Less mortality was found for stomach and lung cancer.

Blair A, Hayes HM Jr. (1982) Mortality patterns among US veterinarians, 1947-1977: an expanded study. Int J Epidemiol. 1982 Dec;11(4):391-7.

Increased risk of esophageal, colon, brain and pancreatic cancer and melanoma in veterinarians in Sweden could not be explained by the socio-economic status of this profession. Occupational exposures to carcinogenic viruses in livestock are potential sources.

Travier N, Gridley G, Blair A, Dosemeci M, Boffetta P. (2003) Cancer incidence among male Swedish veterinarians and other workers of the veterinary industry: a record-linkage study. Cancer Causes Control. 2003 (6):587-93.

Cows are constantly re-impregnated after the birth of the calves by artificial insemination, so that their milk will never stop flowing. The sperm is frozen in "straws" and then introduced by a veterinarian or AI assistant to the animal at the right time, depending on the time of the ovulation cycle. Calves are taken away from their mother soon after birth. Their calves grow up to become dairy cows or are reared for veal. For production of milk and cheese, the mother cow must give birth to as many calves as possible. Female calves grow up to become dairy cows, bulls go to the meat industry. Milk, cheese and meat production are inextricably linked.

Raw egg proteins and raw milk products

Industrially processed food contains a large proportion of liquid chicken egg proteins that in some cases are not sufficiently heated processed. Eggs are released on crushers, egg yolk and white are separated, eggshells and hail cords are removed by filters and the protein product is heated to 56 ° Celsius. In the Netherlands (1983),

20,000 tons of liquid chicken protein was produced for the industry, which was marginally pasteurized sometimes insufficiently heat treated. The confectioner processes a large number of products that contain eggs. This can be the pasteurized proteins, or he processes fresh eggs. The "whites" are collected in a special container. Housewives also sometimes come into contact with raw egg proteins when making cake batter or desserts at home. Or if they whip up the raw egg proteins.

Raw egg proteins are processed in:

SUGAR GLAZE raw egg whites with powdered sugar

ROOM FONDANT raw egg whites with butter, sugar and liqueur

OMELET SIBÉRIEN raw egg whites with sugar

BAVAROIS raw egg whites with sugar, cream, gelatin, fruits

ICE CREAM raw egg whites with sugar, milk and cream.

And also in:

STEAK TARTAR with a raw egg

Raw milk products

Raw milk is milk from cows, sheep, or goats that has not been pasteurized to kill harmful bacteria. This raw, unpasteurized milk can carry dangerous bacteria such as Salmonella, E. coli and Listeria, which are responsible for causing numerous foodborne illnesses.

Employees risks in the poultry industry

———

C arcinogenic viruses are found and cause tumors in chickens and turkeys. A number are carriers and diffusers of these infectious viruses. Virus has been shown in chicken products and eggs, so exposure to humans is universal and almost unavoidable. These viruses are not very contagious, but still have the ability to infect and transform human cells. Antibodies against avian leukemia viruses (ALV) and reticulo endothelial viruses (REV) have been found in blood sera of workers in poultry slaughterhouses. Mortality from cancer has been studied in 20,132 workers in poultry slaughterhouses and processing plants, a group with the highest human exposure to these viruses. The mortality rate among poultry workers has been compared with that of the American population as a whole. Substantially increased risks were observed in poultry workers as a whole or in subgroups, for different cancers: cancer of the mouth and pharynx; pancreas; trachea / bronchus / lung; brain; cervix; lymphocytic leukemia; monocytic leukemia; and tumors of the blood-forming and lymphatic systems. This study provides evidence that a group of people with high exposure to carcinogenic viruses, occurring in poultry, are at a higher risk of death from a number of cancers.

Metayer C, Johnson ES, Rice JC (1998) Nested case-control study of tumors of the hemopoietic and lymphatic systems among workers in the meat industry. Am J Epidemiol 147(8):727-38 https://www.ncbi.nlm.nih.gov/pubmed/9554414

Johnson ES, Ndetan H, Lo KM (2010) Cancer mortality in poultry slaughtering / processing plant workers belonging a union pension fund. Environ Res 110(6):588-94 https://www.ncbi.nlm.nih.gov/pubmed/20541185

Brain cancer is more common in poultry farmers involved in killing chickens. The killing of chickens was accompanied by an almost 6-fold increase in the risk of brain cancer. Workers in poultry slaughterhouses and processing plants often process thousands of chickens daily, come into contact with poultry meat, organs and blood and run the risk of injuries that form a route for viruses and other microbial substances to enter the body. They also work for longer periods in confined spaces, which increases the risk of inhaling microbes. Viruses that are known to cause cancer in poultry can be responsible for the increased incidence of cancer in poultry farmers killing chickens.

Gandhi S, Felini MJ, Nidetan H, Cardarelli K, Jadhav S, Faramawi M, Johnson ES (2014) A pilot case cohort study of brain cancer in poultry and control workers. Nutr Cancer. https://www.ncbi.nlm.nih.gov/pubmed/24564367

Professor Johnson, an epidemiologist at the University of Fort Worth Texas, has published more than 30 articles in scientific journals about increased cancer risks for employees in the meat industry, many of which are specifically for poultry farmers. To definitively link the cancer risk to occupational exposure, he has developed and patented the only test to date that can detect the presence of carcinogenic viruses in the genome of tumor cells of workers with these cancers.

How are consumption animals fed?

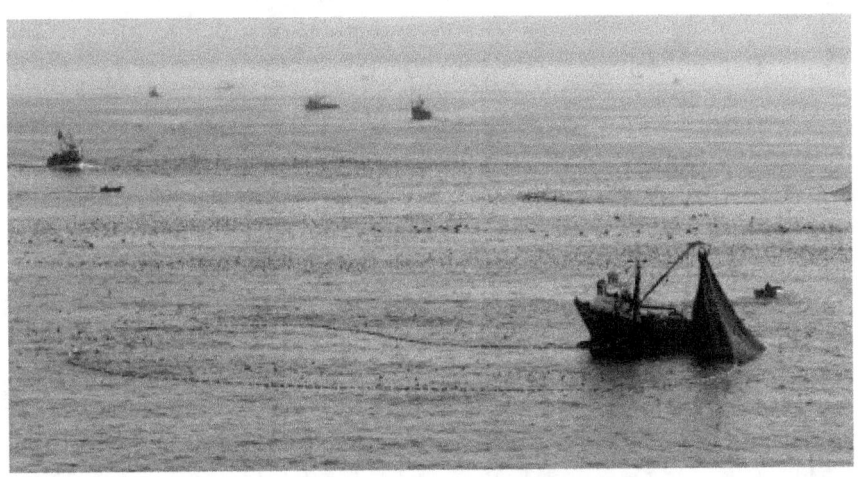

Anchovy from the southeast of the Pacific Ocean is sold as cattle feed to Europe's factory farms. Approximately one third of the total catch is fed to consumption animals, mostly farmed fish, pigs and chickens. European fishermen are obliged to land all by-catches by 2020. In addition to the by-catches, the fish-processing industry also produces a significant amount of reusable waste, such as skins, bones, fish heads and internal organs. Fish meal can be created by hydrolysis of the fish from the by-catches and fish remains, which is a great need. Especially at the fish farms in the Mediterranean. Tuna, salmon, cattle, pigs and chickens grow faster and fatter by fishmeal. More profit can be achieved and the time to slaughter is shortened. For production of fish oil and fishmeal, some 20-30 million tons of fish, anchovies, herring, mackerel and sprat species have been removed from the southeastern Pacific Ocean over the past decades. Consumption on a large scale of small glass eels, and of caviar, fish eggs, is also harmful to fish stocks.

Going back 1000 years in Europe, it was declines in freshwater fish thanks to human pressure which first pushed fishermen out into the oceans in larger numbers. Five hundred years ago, it was the decline of coastal fish that brought deep-sea trawling into existence. A hundred and fifty years ago there was still enough room on the planet. The population growth was still within the carrying capacity of the planet. Today, with the inhabitants of China or India alone equal to those of the entire planet in 1850, humanity has expanded to the point where we are crashing. The earth is overpopulated. As with agriculture, it is not the small businesses that consume the most aid, they are the industrial producers. Worldwide 20 billion is awarded annually. 6.3 billion is spent on subsidies for fuel alone; an extra 8 billion goes to the maintenance of the major ports. Small fishing uses 75% less energy to catch the same volume of fish, more environmentally friendly and with many more people. Abolish these subsidies and industrial fishing suddenly becomes a much less profitable business.

Mega farms with only cows, calves, pigs or chickens feed the animals with soy flour, fish meal and low doses of antibiotics to fatten the animals faster and to gain more profit. This has drastically increased the animal fat content of steak, pork and chicken meat. Welfare diseases such as cardiovascular diseases, increased blood pressure, excess weight and diabetes increase due to food with a high content of saturated animal fat.

What diseases later in life are related to fast food?

———

Increased consumption of energy, animal proteins, animal fats and red meat was produced in different regions of the world after the transition to a more industrialized diet, hamburgers, sugary drinks and fast food in these countries.

With more than 225 million overweight people in 2016, the USA has the largest number of overweight people in the world. The USA also export these unhealthy eating habits around the world. Worse diet is the leading cause of morbidity and mortality in the United States. With an average life expectancy of 78.1 years the United States comes in only at number fifty of the world ranking list, despite being the richest nation on the planet with the most advanced medical technology. The Netherlands is slightly better with an average life expectancy of 79.2 years, less than most other European countries. Even in spite of the nation's alarming high suicide rate Japanese live 82.1 years on average.

Diseases relating to diet are the leading causes of death to the United States. The number of people overweight or obese increased between 1990 and 2016. In the most comprehensive study of US health to date, poor diet was found to be the leading cause of morbidity and mortality, even surpassing smoking. Poor diet contributed to 14 percent, while smoking accounted for 11 percent. Obesity and high blood pressure accounted for 11 and eight percent respectively. The number one cause of death in America is the American diet. High blood pressure by fifty-five, heart attacks at sixty, maybe even cancer at seventy, and so on... For most of the leading causes of death, the science shows that the genes often account for only 10-20% of the risk at most. For example, when people move from low-risk to high-risk countries, their disease rates almost always change to those of the new environment. New diet, new diseases. But the reverse is also true. If we're eating the Standard American Diet and switch to a diet higher in whole plant foods, such as fruits and vegetables, this may lower your risk.

Cancer is now the most common cause of death in Western Europe, more often than chronic obstructive pulmonary disease (COPD) and cardiovascular disease and diabetes (IHD). While mortality rates for COPD and IHD are declining due to improved health care, mortality rates for cancer have increased. Our Western eating habits and addiction to animal proteins in the form of ground beef, hamburgers and all kinds of meat products are the cause of the increase in cancer. The consumption of animal fats and proteins has increased considerably since the last century. The production of meat (products), poultry, pork and other meat tripled between 1980 and 2010 and is likely to double again by 2050. At present, 70 billion farm animals are being bred annually for food. In 2050 there will be 500 million more cattle, 200 million more pigs, 1 billion more sheep and goats and 18 billion extra poultry than in 2005.

As we get older, we notice which unhealthy lifestyle habits have taken possession of us. The body constantly renews itself through the ingested diet and within a few years all cells and tissues are constantly being completely rebuilt. With age, the choice of animal or vegetable protein and fat in the daily diet is of great importance for protection against chronic diseases and cancer. Cardiovascular disease, obesity and uncontrolled growth of derailed cells are the result of an excess of animal proteins and fats in the daily diet. The chicken leukemia virus and bovine leukemia virus in our food chain are related to common cancers. The time without symptoms is 50% - 70% of the total growth of a tumor and cancer usually reveals itself at a later age.

In Japan and Korea, large-scale imports of beef and pork began after the Second World War, respectively after the Korean War. In 1970 in Japan and 1990 in Korea a sharp increase in the numbers of colon cancer was observed. Consumption of fried beef (eg shabu-shabu, Korean yukhoe and Japanese yukke) became very popular in both countries. A specific meat factor, presumably one or more thermo-resistant potential carcinogenic bovine viruses (for example polyoma, papilloma or single-stranded DNA viruses), can contaminate the beef and lead to latent infections in the intestinal tract.

Zur Hausen H (2012) Red meat consumption and cancer: reasons for suspect involvement or bovine infectious factors in colorectal cancer. Int J Cancer. 2012 Jun 1; 130 (11): 2475-83

https://www.ncbi.nlm.nih.gov/pubmed/22212999

Increased consumption of energy, animal fat and Red meat has occurred in East Asia in recent decades. Data on breast cancer, colon, prostate, esophagus and stomach cancer mortality rates for China (1988-2000), Hong Kong (1960-2006), Japan (1950-2006), Korea (1985-2006) and Singapore (1963- 2006) were obtained from the WHO. In the selected countries (except breast cancer in Hong Kong), a noticeable increase in mortality rates of breast, colon and prostate cancer and a decreasing decrease in esophageal and gastric cancer in the study periods were observed. For example, the annual percentage increase in mortality in breast cancer was 5.5% for the period 1985-1993 in Korea and the mortality rates for prostate cancer increased from 1958 to 1993 in Japan by 3.2% per year. These changes in cancer mortality followed ~ 10 years after the transition to more industrially prepared food, hamburgers, sugary drinks and fast food in these countries.

Zhang J, Dhakai IB, Zhao Z, Li L (2012) Trends in mortality from cancers of the breast, colon, prostate, esophagus, and stomach in East Asia: role of nutrition transition. Eur J Cancer Prev 2012 Sep; 21 (5): 480-9 https://www.ncbi.nlm.nih.gov/pubmed/22357483

Mortality rates for prostate cancer have increased dramatically (25x) in Japan after the Second World War. After the war the consumption of milk increased by 20x, from meat 9x and from eggs 7x. Milk contains large amounts of estrogens plus proteins and saturated fats. The recent increase in its use is likely to be the cause of the surge of prostate cancer in Japan.

Ganmaa D, Li XM, Qin LQ et al. The experience of Japan as a clue to the etiology of testicular and prostatic cancers. Med Hypotheses. 2003 May; 60 (5): 724-30

https://www.ncbi.nlm.nih.gov/pubmed/12710911

The inhabitants of Tuvalu, Fiji, Samoa and the Cook Islands are massively overweight. According to the World Health Organization (WHO), nine of the world's ten thickest countries belong to the Pacific Islands. Tonga (4th, 90.8%), Samoa (6th, 80.4%) and USA (9th, 74.1%). Up to 95 percent of the adult population is overweight in some countries. The number of people with obesity, extremely overweight, varies from 35 to 50 percent. The Cook Islands (90.9% overweight) are in third place in the world ranking. Slightly more than half of the population suffers from obesity. Inexpensive factory processed food has replaced the original diet of fresh fish and vegetables. Fresh fish is relatively expensive, with this money you can buy multiple hamburger meals. A bottle of cola is cheaper here than a bottle of water. 75% of the women on Samoa are extremely overweight.

https://youtu.be/RSwpX15ZNcA

How great is the loss of animal and plant species?

———

- In the last 50 years homo sapiens has wiped out 60% of mammals, birds, fish and reptiles in the wild
- Humankind has destroyed 83% of all mammals and half of plants since the dawn of civilization.
- Wildlife hunting in tropical forests reduces bird and mammal populations.

Our ancestors have likely consumed bushmeat, wild animals killed for food. During the 20th century, however, commercial hunting using firearms and wire snares to supply logging and oil exploration concessions along new roadway networks has dramatically increased the catch in Central African forests. Annually, it is estimated that 579 million wild animals are caught and consumed in the Congo basin, equaling 4.5 million tons of bushmeat, with the addition of a possible 5 million tons of wild mammalian meat from the Amazon basin. Tropical lowland forest habitat contains the world's greatest terrestrial biodiversity and may therefore harbor a reservoir of zoonotic pathogens. The wildlife trade in general generates in excess one billion direct and indirect contacts between humans and domesticated animals annually. The broad range of tissue and fluid exposures associated with the bush meat industry's hunting and butchering may take these wildlife interactions especially risky. In Africa, as many as 30 different species of primates are also hunted and processed by the bushmeat industry.

- The increase in meat products and dairy production in the West could only be achieved with artificial insemination of livestock and the animals unilaterally fattening with soy flour, corn and fish meal.

- One billion people suffer from hunger, while 70 billion animals are fattened and eaten every year.
- During the ice ages the Cro-Magnon man was forced to eat more meat because there were fewer grains, fruit, nuts and seeds. Will modern man start eating more fruit and vegetables now that the earth is warming up?

We can no longer ignore the impact of current unsustainable production models. If we start eating less meat, the farmers can gradually switch from intensive livestock farming to agriculture

Benítez-López A, Alkemade R, Schipper AM et al. The impact of hunting on tropical mammal and bird populations. Science 2017 356(6334):180-183

Population growth to seven, eight or nine billion causes food shortages, diseases and climate changes due to intensive meat production. The large number of animals locked up for meat consumption is the perfect system as a source for pathogenic viruses such as highly pathogenic influenza, corona virus and leukemia virus. The human race is moving in the same direction as the species that we have seen disappearing.

How do we make a greenhouse of the earth?

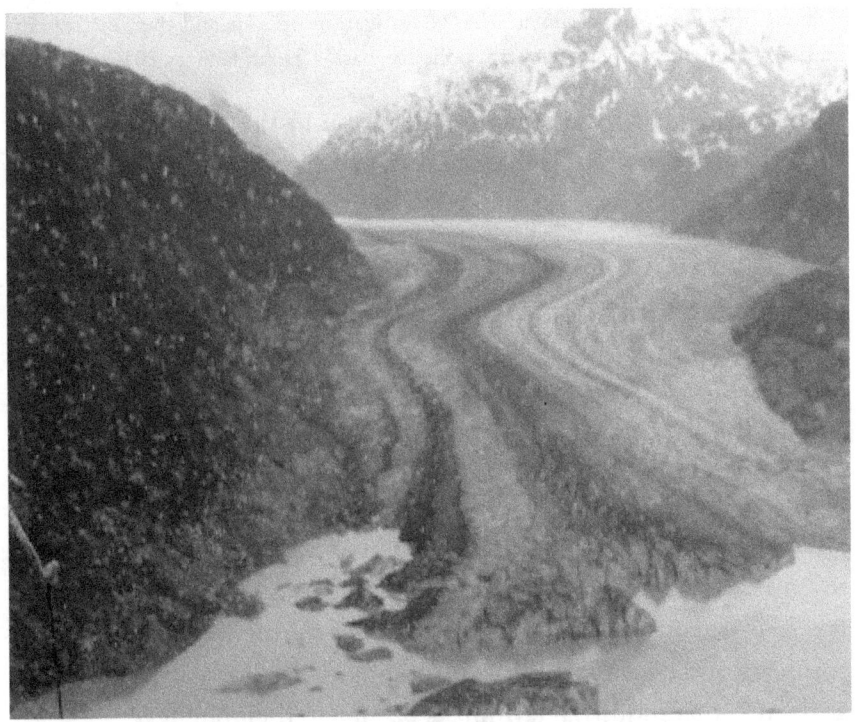

- Every year the glaciers in Alaska become hundreds of meters shorter by melting the ice. https://youtu.be/HY671_UR-qo
- In the USA, cattle emit approximately 5.5 million m3 of methane, a greenhouse 25 times more potent than CO2.

The fast-growing meat industry produces more greenhouse gases than the exhaust gases from all car traffic on earth. Melting glaciers are the result of this. Meat, milk and eggs in our food contribute more to the climate change in the world than the exhaust fumes of our fleet. Livestock farming accounts for at least 14.5% and, according to some studies, even 51% of man-made greenhouse gases. In the USA cattle emit approximately 5.5 million m3 of methane - a greenhouse gas that is 25 times more potent than CO_2.

CE Delft, Fraunhofer Institute for Systems and Innovation Research and LEI Wageningen. Behavioural climate change mitigation options and their appropriate inclusion in quantitative longer-term policy scenarios. Delft, January 2012

All life depends on the oceans. Circulation in the North Atlantic has slowed to the lowest level in centuries. The slowdown of the Gulf Stream devastates fisheries and will lead to a rise in sea levels.

Large amounts of nitrogen from fertilizer and manure are distributed annually over agricultural land. No doubt that it increases crop yield, but plants do not absorb it completely, so that more fertilizer and animal waste is added than the plants need. Only a fraction of what is applied to the soil ends up in the crops. The rest flows to our rivers.

Nitrogen and phosphorus levels, dead organisms are increasing in the Gulf of Mexico, the Rhône Delta, the North Sea, the Baltic Sea and the Adriatic Sea. Oxygen levels fall in these coastal waters. Dead Zone takes us on an eye-opening investigative journey across the globe, focussing on a dozen iconic species one-by-one and looking in each case at the role that industrial farming is playing in their plight.

This is a wake-up call for us all, laying bare the myths that prop up factory farming before exploring what we can do to save the planet with healthy food (Phillip Lymbery. 2017).

How we made a desert of the land on earth?

———

A llan Savory. https://youtu.be/vpTHi7O66pI

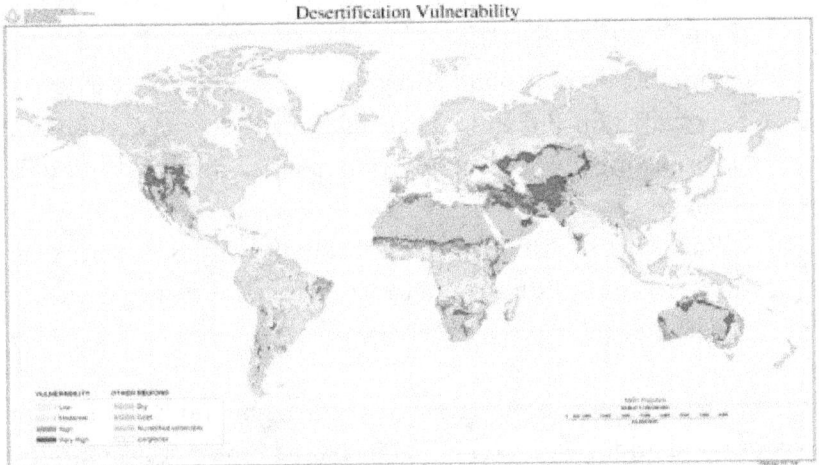

Desertification Vulnerability

Desertification on 2/3 of the land on earth

- When humans mastered fire, language and developed weapons like spears and axes, they were formidable predators. This was especially the case in the grasslands where their prey ran in herds. The grasslands with their deep, water and carbonaceous soils had developed for millions of years thanks to the balance between grazing animals, and the predators that fed with them.
- Modern farming methods contribute significantly to desertification and climate change due to water and air pollution from agriculture and intensive breeding of pigs,

poultry and livestock. By breaking down agricultural land, we are reducing its enormous ability to retain and contain carbon.

- Chemical fertilizers to increase production have killed micro-organisms in the soil, reduced fertility of the soil and the ability to retain water and led to additional flooding. Pesticides used for the treatment of internal parasites in animals have led to the destruction of dung beetles, which are vital for soil renewal.
- Fires break the ground cover in a way that it easily carries away by rain and wind. Huge man-made deserts have arisen. According NASA pictures from space about two thirds of the land is deserted.
- Banks finance the farmers to rent out their pastures for solar panels and windmills and to set up even more megafarms with the aid of electrical energy.

An ever-growing meat production causes drought and hunger in large parts of the world. Fast food and an increase in meat consumption in the West are also being imitated in other parts of the world. Modern agriculture makes an important contribution to desertification and climate change due to water and air pollution from agriculture and intensive breeding of pigs, poultry and livestock. By demolishing agricultural land, we reduce the enormous ability of land to hold carbon.

Abolition of Slavery

A fter the Spanish flu (Influenza H1N1 pandemic originated from the poultry industry), which ruled from 1918 to 1920, due to pandemic measures the economic situation was bad, schools and resorts were closed. An economic crisis also followed in the interwar period. After World War II, the United Nations was established to define land and human rights. Later human slavery was abolished.

Will there be an economic crisis with many deaths after the second wave of Coronaviruses from 2019 to 2021 (pandemic originated from the meat industry)? The climate crisis seems inevitable and there is a great loss of plant and animal species. There are already more bats than people. Will this mammalian species prevail or will humans gain insight and abolish the slavery of wild life and food animals?

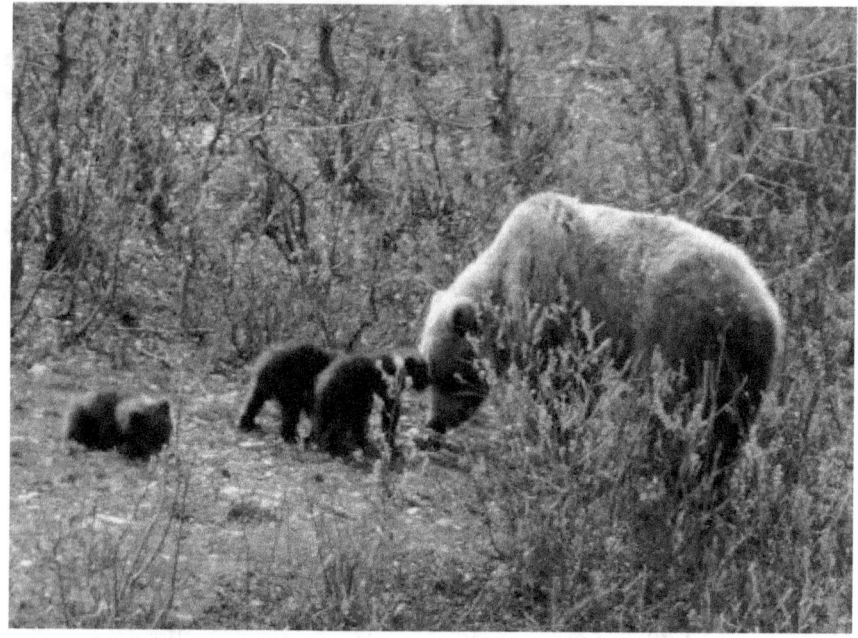

Boar with three youngs in Denali tundra wilderness

All mammals must have the opportunity to care for their offspring themselves.

Artificial insemination of livestock and factory farming of cows, goats, pigs, sheep and rabbits is a gross violation of this fundamental mammalian right. All mammals have a basis of life and the right to live without cruel treatment and prolonged detention.

Grasslands and grazing animals have an enormous ability to hold carbon. Agriculture can produce better vegetable and fruit as food for humans than the corn and soybeans with which we now fatten and confine the animals in factory farms to be eaten by humans.

Contraception

To put an end to the abuses in the Kempen that physician Ferdinand Peeters encountered in his daily practice, he went in search of a means by which the woman, for the sake of life, could arrange her own fertility. The contraceptive pill Enovid put on the market by the American biologist Gregory Pincus in 1957 still had too many side effects and was only admitted as a remedy for painful periods. In 1959, Dr. Peeters started a series of clinical tests with a hormone preparation offered by the German company Schering AG from his lab in the Sint-Elizabeth hospital in Turnhout. For six months, Dr. Peeters and his assistants Reimond Oeyen and Marcel Van Roy tested the preparation on fifty Kempen women for whom even more children posed a major health risk. After numerous experiments to find the right (more than half lower) dose of the two hormones (progestin and estrogen), in 1960 Peeters explained the findings to Schering in Berlin. The results were amazing. Not one of the women became pregnant and there were hardly any side effects. After Peeters' preparation (SH 639) was found to be safe and efficient in the United States, Japan and the United Kingdom as well, Schering markets the Anovlar pill in January 1961. Pincus tacitly acknowledged the superiority of Peeters' pill by halving the dose of Enovid in July 1961. In the end, it was Pincus who took the credit and (erroneously) went down in history all over the world as the inventor of the contraceptive pill. For fear of being robbed by the Church, however, the very Catholic Peeters did not give much publicity to his invention. Moreover, the pioneering research of a 'rural doctor' also aroused a lot of contempt among jealous professors from the KUL where Peeters was also active.

- For centuries, sheep intestine and since 1844 Goodyear rubber has been used as a contraceptive.
- The pill, IVF and artificial insemination brought the breakthrough in the middle of the twentieth century.
- The German company Schering AG put the Anovlar pill on the market in January 1961.
- The pill proved to be a particularly powerful emancipatory agent, both in America and in Europe. The pill radically changed the balance of power between men and women - and with it the entire society.
- By population control, the population growth decreased, while prosperity increased the dependency of the elderly decreased.

The discovery of the pill was a great revolution. For the first time in human history, sexual intercourse and reproduction could be technically and artificially separated. The enormous commercial success was blinding, both for medicine and for theology. And everyone tried to outdo the other in giving good justification for birth control. Contraception caused a radical break with the lives of all previous generations and civilizations. Legal abortion has since been introduced, the number of divorces has increased spectacularly, euthanasia has been advocated if life is no longer experienced as meaningful. The family as the basis of church and society has crumbled into all sorts of free living together. All forms of sexuality are then openly discussed. The emergence of gays, Me Too for unwanted intimacies, sexual intimidation and rape, incest and pedophilia, gender change of transgender people, genital mutilation in other cultures. The sexual abstinence of the celibacy also had its problems such as pedophilia in priests.

Yet the balance of sudden sexual freedom is positive overall, thanks to the increased emancipation of women and the awareness of sexual problems and liberties that have been hidden for years. There are more and more women in managerial positions. There have been Queens for quite some time, but now women have also become ministers and president. We are still waiting for the first woman as pope, now that the woman has also been admitted to church.

In the metropolis of Ghuangzhou (the former Canton), our guide pointed us to a female Buddha in the largest temple.

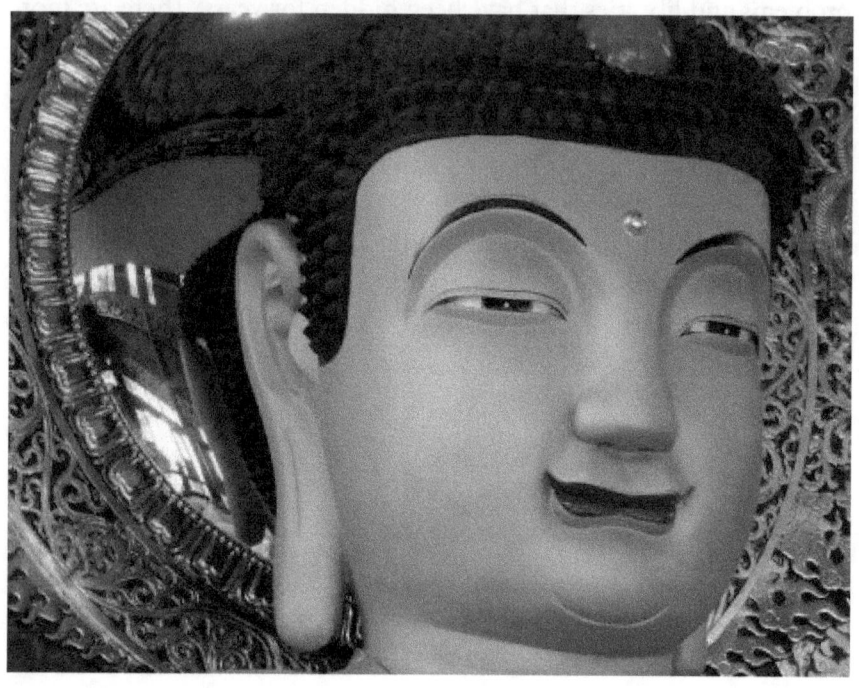

What does the sun give us?

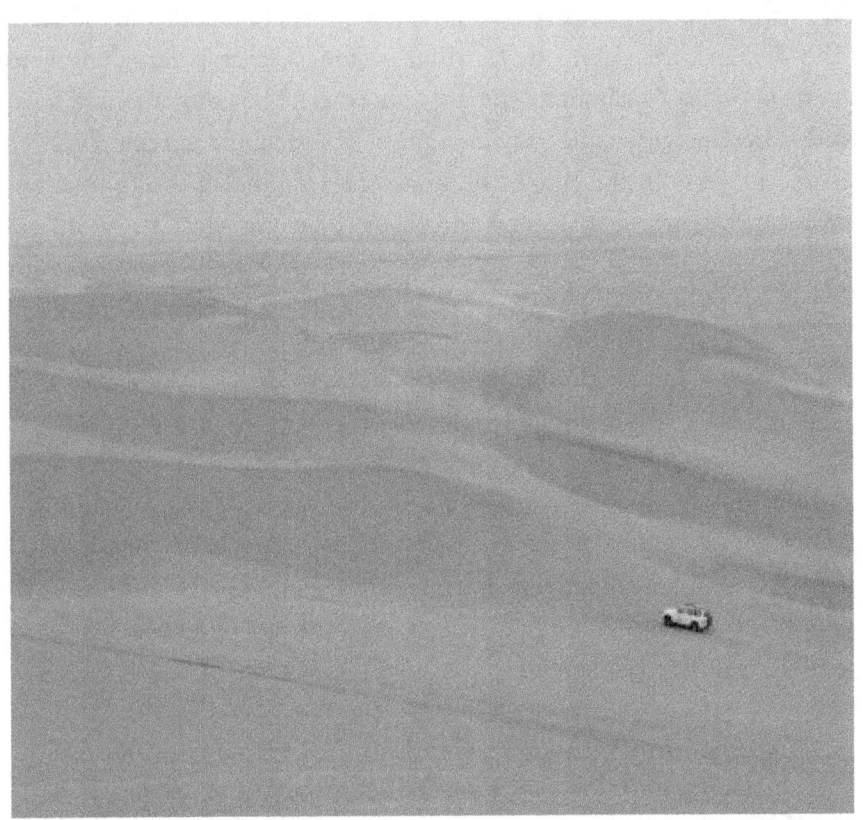

The Namid desert

In 54 minutes, drops to the earth the amount of solar energy that the whole world consumes in one year. All free renewable energy. Only it is in the wrong place at the wrong time in the wrong form. If we turn all that energy into hydrogen on a daily basis, the scarcity of energy is immediately over. All this energy can be stored in the form of hydrogen and transported through the gas network and in liquid form by ship.

Every day that we do nothing with the storage of solar and wind energy here and there in the Netherlands and in the deserts is a lost day. It's not really complicated, we just have to make the right decisions.

We will be saying goodbye not only to fossil fuels, but also to biofuels. The demand for palm oil has risen so much what is largely due to western policy to stimulate the use of biofuels. The cosmetics and food industries are also major customers. Fires has become increasingly fierce in recent years in the Brazilian Amazon forest and in the Indonesian tropical rainforests of Borneo and Papua New Guinea. The 'slash and burn' method (felling and burning) is used to cultivate natural land for palm plantations. Hydrogen as prime energy source is the solution.

- The Namib desert at Lüderitz, a port on the Atlantic Ocean on the south-west coast of Namibia, is one of the sunniest places in the world. This desert is 200 km wide and extends 2000 km from Angola in the North to the Orange River in the South along the Atlantic Ocean. In this 81,000 km2 a suitable area for energy production can be found. A combination of solar panels and hydrogen gas production with transport to the sea can offer economic benefits to poor Namibia. https://youtu.be/a04JKguARZA

- Let Groningen earn from the transition to hydrogen gas. The Netherlands already has an extensive gas network from Groningen to the rest of the Netherlands. This natural gas network can be used for hydrogen gas transport without too much adaptation so that most domestic and industrial connections can use hydrogen gas for heating, cooking and industrial use.
- Veendam has the first larger hydrogen plant in the Netherlands that uses solar power. It is an important step in Groningen's mission to develop into the hydrogen province of the Netherlands. Renewable energy from the electricity

grid and 5,000 solar panels on the site provide green electricity to the plant, which can convert one megawatt of sustainable electricity into hydrogen. A hydrogen industry in Groningen can supply the large amounts of energy that will be lost when the oil and gas era is closed. Hydrogen can be stored in empty salt caverns on the Energy Stock site. If all the salt caverns on the site are filled with hydrogen, that will be enough to heat all the houses in the Netherlands for several weeks.

- Researchers from the University of Waterloo in Canada have developed a new fuel cell that lasts at least ten times longer than current technology. These fuel cells can produce electricity from the chemical reaction, when hydrogen and oxygen are combined to make water, and will therefore be much cheaper. If these fuel cells are mass-produced, they will be able to power hydrogen-gas hybrid vehicles. http://www.uwaterloo.ca

- Canadian engineers have found a way to produce hydrogen relatively easily and cheaply. By injecting oxygen into the tar sands, the temperature in the soil appears to rise. As a result, hydrogen gas is released from the oil, which can be separated from other gases by special membrane filters. The procedure works in tar sands, but also exhausted and discarded oil fields: wherever there is still oil in the ground that can be heated, leading to the formation of hydrogen gas. Even with oil fields that are still in use, this technique can be used. A polluting fossil resource can thus be given a new lease of life and produce the energy carrier of the future. Hydrogen production is a cost-effective alternative to energy production from oil fields and tar sands. By placing hydrogen filter membranes in the production sources, only the hydrogen is extracted and undesirable by-products such as carbon dioxide diode and methane remain in the soil.

- The existing infrastructure and distribution channels around the oil fields would suffice, keeping production costs low. At the moment it costs about 2 dollars to produce a kilo of H2, but with the new method that would only be 10 to 50 cents. The necessary oxygen can be produced on site. This requires no more than 5 percent of the energy produced.

- The oil sands deposits in Western Canada not only represent a vast store of hydrocarbons (oil) that can be converted into fuel and petrochemicals but also a vast hydrogen store – a super clean valuable energy vector and chemical feedstock. Oil sands reservoirs have low energy and emissions intensities, hydrogen production is a viable alternative for energy production from heavy oil and oil sands reservoirs by using in situ gasification technology. Gasification reactions, together with the water-gas shift reaction, enable the generation of hydrogen from both bitumen and water within the oil sands reservoir. With hydrogen separation membranes in the production wells, other products from the reactions remain in the reservoir.

Chemical preparation of hydrogen from sodium borohydride

Sodium boron hydride (NaBH 4) is a chemical compound from which hydrogen can be extracted. In combination with fuel cells, electricity can be produced safely and with only water as a residual product. The material is a white powder and a well-known ingredient of washing powders. A Dutch inventor brought sodium boron hydride into contact with very pure water and a catalyst. The result: more than 95% of the theoretically feasible amount of hydrogen is actually extracted. A great success that has since been patented and is being further developed, in collaboration with Technical University Delft. You do need water without ions. It is transported to the filling station in granular form. A machine there makes ultrapure water from tap water. The ultrapure water is then mixed with the sodium boron hydride, creating a pumpable slurry. The 'slurry' - called H2Fuel - is then filled up, just like you fill up with petrol. A truck, with only 350 litres of sodium boron hydride can go up and down to Barcelona without refuelling. The H2Fuel process, with a very high yield, has already been validated by TNO (www.h2fuel.com[1]).

H2Fuel, a sodium-borohydride compound, is the carrier of hydrogen. The chemical name is $NaBH_4$ (powder) and can be stored indefinitely under normal atmospheric conditions. To release the hydrogen, Ultra Pure Water (UPW = fully pure H_2O) and a little dilute hydrochloric acid are added in a certain ratio and the hydrogen molecules of both the $NaBH_4$ and H_2O are released. A total of 8H. This high yield of hydrogen molecules is only possible with the use of UPW (patented). With this hydrogen, electricity and / or heat can be produced via a fuel cell.

On sea-going vessels osmosis allows UPW to extract fully pure water from seawater and space is available for this type of power plant.

A Hyundai NEXO is equipped with a 156-liter compression tank (700 bar) with hydrogen gas and has a range of 666 km. The high vehicle weight (1814 kg) comes at the expense of acceleration. With a 60-liter normal tank with sodium borohydride powder slurry, a hydrogen car can be much lighter and have a range of 700 km (2.5 times larger with the same amount of hydrogen).

The drive system of the Hyundai Nexo delivers a power of 135 kW (184 hp) and with a full tank of hydrogen you can cover approximately 580

---

1. http://www.h2fuel.com

kilometres. Taking H2 fuel from the farmer and revaluing the residual liquid will be possible. Great figures for daily use.

A grant project to speed up the chemical preparation of hydrogen would be great. A greenhouse complex in the Westland wants to be able to produce energy-neutral fruit and vegetables all year round with the help of a hydrogen power plant. Some vans are also converted into hydrogen cars and can refuel at the greenhouse complex and have the residual liquid here upgraded.

Vertical agriculture and horticulture require a lot of heat, light and space to produce strawberries, lettuce, cauliflower, peppers, grapes and also tropical fruit such as pineapples all year round. Here too, such a power plant with fuel cells can be used. Farmers can give their warehouses a new destination. With local production with a greater supply and diversity, the current supply of fruit and vegetables over the equator will be able to decrease.

What about the recent increase in cancer?

Bowel Cancer

An increased risk of colorectal cancer has long been shown for the consumption of undercooked red meat. Fish and chicken do not increase this risk, although comparable or even higher concentrations of potentially cancer-causing chemicals are released during roasting or frying. In Japan and Korea, beef and pork were imported on a large scale after the Second World War and the Korean War. A strong increase in the number of patients with colon cancer was observed after 1970 in Japan and after 1990 in Korea. The consumption of undercooked beef (eg, Shabu-shabu, Korean Yukhoe and Japanese Yukke) became very popular in both countries.

Bovine leukemia virus as a source of colon cancer

A specific beef factor, probably one or more heat-resistant carcinogenic bovine viruses (for example, polyoma, papilloma or bovine leukemia virus BLV) can infect the beef and cause latent and persistent intestinal infections after human consumption (Zur Hausen H).

Polyoma viruses in hamburgers

In chopped beef samples three types of polyoma virus have been shown, which are resistant to BBQ temperatures and are carcinogenic to their natural hosts. Animal viruses are frequently found in meat products and can cause colon cancer in humans. The papilloma and polyoma viruses in particular are resistant to medium-heated steak tartar, in which the central parts of the meat are not heated above 40 - 70 degrees Celsius. These viruses endure 80 degrees Celsius for 30 minutes without losing too much of their ability to cause infections. These viruses are also insufficiently inactivated during the pasteurization of dairy products.

Acid-resistant bacteria and stomach cancer

Two Australian GPs realized that mycobacteria (acid-solid organisms) can survive the acidic environment of the stomach, which other pathogenic bacteria cannot. They discovered one of the most important human pathogens, Helicobacter pylori, which are capable of causing severe stomach inflammatory disease. It was then discovered that these microbes cause gastric carcinoma.

Lichtman MA A Bacterial Cause of Cancer: An Historical Essay. Oncologist. 2017 May;22(5):542-548

https://www.ncbi.nlm.nih.gov/pubmed/28432224

Zhang J, Dhakai IB, Zhao Z, Li L (2012) Trends in mortality from cancers of the breast, colon, prostate, oesophagus, and stomach in East Asia: role of nutrition transition. Eur J Cancer Prev 2012 Sep;21(5):480-9

https://www.ncbi.nlm.nih.gov/pubmed/22357483

Zur Hausen H (2012) Red meat consumption and cancer: reasons to suspect involvement of bovine infectious factors in colorectal cancer. Int J Cancer.130(11):2475-83

https://www.ncbi.nlm.nih.gov/pubmed/22212999

Breast Cancer

People are exposed to carcinogenic viruses that often occur in animals in the food chain, such as laying hens, eggs, broiler chickens and dairy cows. The Avian Leukemia Virus (ALV) and Bovine Leukemia Viruses (BLV) are RNA viruses and have been shown in breast cancer cells.

BOVINE LEUKEMIA VIRUS in breast cancer cells

Breast cancer and ovarian cancer were rare in Japan, compared with other countries. The mortality rates, however, are increasing. After the Second World War changes in lifestyle took place in Japan. In the past 50 years (1947-1997), mortality rates of breast and ovarian cancer increased 2- and 4-fold, and the respective intake of milk, meat and eggs increased 20, 10 and 7-fold. The increase in death rates from breast cancer and ovarian cancer could be attributed to the increased consumption of animal nutrition, which occurred after 1945. Milk, dairy products and eggs are probably the cause of this (Buehring). Cows are often infected with bovine leukemia virus (BLV), a carcinogenic virus that can be transferred from the cow to the calf via the milk or during birth. Most infected cattle seem healthy and the infection is persistent. Consumption of non-pasteurized dairy products, or cheese made from raw milk, or insufficiently heated beef at the BBQ can transmit this infectious virus to humans. About 38% of the cattle, 84% of the dairy herd, and 100% of factory farm herds in the US are infected with BLV. Less than 5% of these cattle get leukemia. With this condition the animals are not admitted to the US consumer market. The BLV virus circulates with the white blood cells through the blood of infected cattle. The BLV virus also infects the mammary gland cells of the cows and infected cells are found in cow's milk (Lanou AJ). Pasteurization of cow's milk makes the BLV ineffective.

Buehring GC (2015) has shown that 39% of people in a San Francisco Bay Area have antibodies against BLV in the blood, which is an indication of exposure to BLV. Almost all cow's milk contains BLV bovine leukemia virus. In a study of 213 women, BLV-related DNA was found in breast tissue of women with a diagnosis of breast cancer, not in breast tissue of women without history of breast cancer (Buehring).

Ovarian and fallopian tube cancer in laying hens

Ovarian cancer often occurs in laying hens (Frederickson TN). For this reason, they are usually slaughtered after the first leg year. In poultry farms, laying hens do not become older than 24 months. Avian Leukemia Virus (leucosis) is a retrovirus that infects large parts of the modern poultry farms and caused a lot of economic damage. The virus is present in chickens and eggs. Man is exposed to this. RNA viruses are single-stranded proteins that do not accurately divide. When RNA viruses divide within a host cell, they make many copies that differ from the original. Some of these copy differences increase their genetic variation and survival chances in the host. Therefore, although it is often possible to prevent a DNA virus infection with a sustainable vaccine, it is very difficult, if not impossible, to make a sustainable vaccine for an RNA virus, especially the RNA retroviruses. This also makes RNA viruses very difficult to treat with medicines.

Mice also infect the grain stocks with a virus that is closely related to breast cancer viruses (Stewart TH). Free-range chickens are often kept outside, so that the risk of contamination due to the contamination of food on the ground by mouse droppings is greater. In the winter months, mice often go to poultry farms to look for food. Virus spreading mice; contamination of cereals, chicken feeds and poultry; transfer by infected chickens from viruses to the eggs; processing of raw, insufficiently heated protein in confectionery products; this is how the ALV virus arrives in humans (Pham TD).

Raw proteins often contain leukemia virus (ALV and BLV)

Breast and colon cancer are not caused by breathing bad air. A causal relationship will be found earlier for pathogens in our diet. Animal proteins in milk and dairy products, in meat products and in egg proteins carry carcinogenic viruses. Improved laboratory techniques provide increasing evidence. A total of 22,788 persons with lactose intolerance were examined, who did not use milk products, and compared with people who did use milk products. The risk of lung, breast and colon cancer appeared to be significantly reduced in the group that did not use milk products. The risk of lung, breast and colon cancer appeared to be significantly reduced in the group that did not use milk products.

Ji J, Sundquist J, Sundquist K Lactose intolerance and reduced risk of lung, breast and ovarian cancers: aetiological clues from a population-based study in Sweden. Br J Cancer. 2015 Jan 6; 112 (1): 149-52

https://www.ncbi.nlm.nih.gov/pubmed/25314053

Breast cancer and ovarian cancer are they ZOONOSES?

The observation that chickens may be infected with a closely related form of mouse breast cancer virus (MMTV) may be of epidemiological significance for human breast cancer. Chickens and eggs can be infected by mice and in turn pass the virus on to people. The successful infection of human cells by MMTV has already been demonstrated (Indik S 2007). MMTV can infect human cell cultures and this finding provides a possible explanation for the discovery of MMTV in patients with breast cancer. The numbers of breast cancer that occur in humans vary geographically. No environmental factor could explain this variation. The highest incidence of breast cancer worldwide occurs in countries where Mus domesticus is the native or imported type of house mouse.

Stewart TH, Sage RD, Stewart AF, Cameron DW (2000) Breast cancer incidence highest in the range of one species of house mouse, Mus domesticus. Br J Cancer. 82(2):446-51.

https://www.ncbi.nlm.nih.gov/pubmed/10646903

Breast stem cells

Women who have remained childless have immature mammary cells with stem cell activity. When these cells become infected with carcinogenic virus, this infection leads to uncontrolled cell division. In the twentieth century, breast cancer was also called "the nuns disease." Full-term pregnancies reduce the risk of breast cancer and the higher the number of pregnancies, the greater this protection. The risk of breast cancer decreases by 7% after every full-term pregnancy. Women who have given birth to children have a 30% lower risk than childless women. Stem cells in the mammary gland are only developed after the first full-term pregnancy. Immature gland cells possess stem cell properties. The stem cell properties cause uncontrolled cell division at the time of infection or other forms of cell damage. The presence of breast cancer in the woman is closely related to her age. Breast cancer is most common in childless women and women around menopause. The biological regression of women begins around the time of menopause and is accompanied by a reduction of immune function of body cells. Reduced cell defenses can lead to the proliferation of infected mammary cells.

Lifestyle medicine

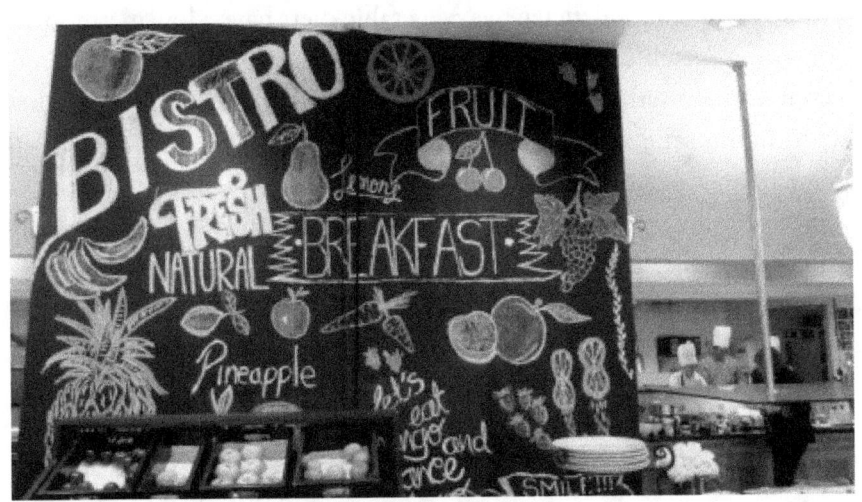

How to become healthy 100 years old

We eat everything that tastes good. If it is cheap and tasty, it also accelerates chronic disease and tumor formation. This is how our food system works. The raw materials for factory preparation are limited. Soy, corn, eggs, refined sugars, animal proteins and trans fats. These are the main ingredients that the largest food companies use to make the food that is all around us. It is not that these big companies do not care. In fact, it is difficult for them to do something else. In parts of the world with less chemical agriculture, less factory food processing, mortality from cancer is lower. Fruits and vegetables contain more bio-active substances.

- Fruits and vegetables make bio-active substances that delay the growth and propagation of intruders.

Plant-based nutrition works life-extending

Voluntary diet through starvation will probably never gain much popularity as a life-prolonging strategy and is risky in connection with the development of deficiencies. Vegetable diets have a low methionine content. Vegetable proteins - especially those from vegetables or nuts - contain less methionine than animal proteins. Several animal studies with methionine restricted diet have shown inhibition of cancer cell growth and prolonged healthy life span in experimental animals. American researchers have looked at 30 years of nutrition data among 130,000 people. They found a reduced risk of premature death in those who ate more vegetable protein and a higher risk in those who ate more animal protein. Each increase of 3% more vegetable proteins in the diet reduced the risk of death, by whatever cause, during the period under review by 10%. A link was also shown with a 12% lower risk of death from cardiovascular disease. But a 10% higher share of animal proteins in the diet led to a 2% higher risk of death and 8% higher chance of dying of a heart problem (Song M).

Plant-based food is not boring and one-sided. Exotic fruits, herbs, soya and vegetables can very well replace all meat and meat products in supermarkets. On the land, 250,000 different varieties of plants can be grown and in oceans there are another 20,000 different species, including seaweed, rich in omega-3 oils. The countries of the southern hemisphere could also make a larger contribution to this. The recipe is still in its infancy.

Animal proteins and vegetable proteins from the oceans are healthier than animal proteins from intensive livestock farming. The oceans offer a good choice of anchovies, mussels, oysters, squid, herring, mackerel, cod, sprat, sole, crabs, lobsters, shrimps and even wild tuna and salmon.

The human body defends against invading bacteria, spores and yeast cells, with the help of antibodies, white blood cells, macrophages and

T-cells. The body is unable to produce antioxidants such as beta-carotene, vitamin C and is unable to make vegetable bio-active substances.

Unnatural nutrition is the cause of deficits and chronic diseases. Fast food, many meat products and little fruit and vegetables weaken the natural defenses. The question remains how a revolution in public opinion can be achieved in order to massively switch exclusively to natural food with supplementing necessary supplements for existing shortages.

Oatmeal flakes

Whole grain is an important source of antioxidants and bioactive compounds such as phenols, flavenoids and carotenoids. Flavenoids work very well as an antioxidant and prevent the conversion of calories into fat. Thus they also have a protective effect on the blood vessels. The majority of the health-promoting compounds of whole grain are present in the germ and bran.

Vitamin C

Not so long ago during the great voyages of discovery, it has already been discovered that vitamin C deficiencies arise due to lack of fresh fruit and vegetables. This gave the sailors scurvy with internal bleeding, which usually resulted in death. Vitamin C is necessary for the construction of connective tissue proteins. Deficient production of these connective tissue proteins weakens the blood vessels with bleeding as a result. Due to the frequent use of pesticides in agriculture, the content of bioactive antibodies in fruit and vegetables has been reduced, as a result of which our defense against cell infections is even more affected.

Vitamin D

Sufficient vitamin D increases bone density, which means less chance of bone fractures. Vitamin D is not really a vitamin, but the precursor of the powerful steroid hormone calcitrol, which has widespread actions throughout the body. Several studies have shown that vitamin D deficiency increases the risk of developing cancer and that avoiding a deficiency and adding vitamin D supplements can be an economical and safe way to reduce the incidence of cancer and the prognosis and result of cancer treatment. Vitamin D is a fat-soluble vitamin and is sold as pearl capsules. Vitamin supra D3 forte capsules (Bayer) contain 20 mcg equivalent to 800 IU. If a deficiency has been established, at least 2 pearls per day should be taken.

Curcuma

Curcuma is the spice that turns curry powder yellow. In areas where this herb is eaten daily, a number of cancer diseases that are very common in Western Europe are less common.

Numerous nutrients from plants, one of the best known is curcum (from turmeric, curry), protect against damage to the chromosomes of cells in the body. Malignant growth, in general, is due to DNA attack upon exposure to chemicals, radiation, or viruses that take possession of the host cell's DNA. Curcuma protects against cell DNA damage and helps clean up affected cells. Infected or damaged cells are now seen as abnormal and are removed from the body by growth inhibition and the death of the infected cell. Herbs and fruits often contain the nutrients that fast food lacks.

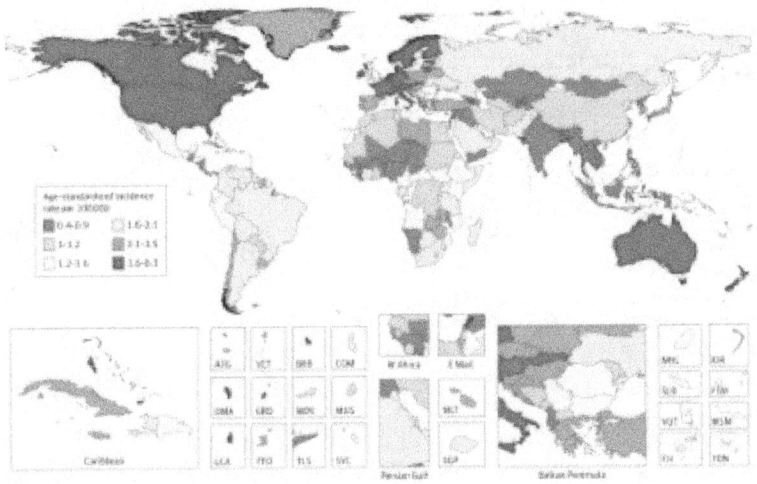

Andrew J. Cowan, Christine Allen, Aleksandra Barac et al. Global burden of multiple myeloma: A systematic analysis for the global burden of disease study 2016. JAMA Oncol 2018 Sep 1;4(9):1221-1227

Total cancer mortality is much lower in India than in Western countries. American men get 23 times more prostate cancer than men in India. Americans 8 and 14 times more likely to develop melanoma, 10 to 11 times more colon cancer, 9 times more uterine cancer, 7-17 times more lung cancer, 7-8 times more bladder cancer, 5 times more breast cancer and 9 to 12 times more often kidney cancer than in India. This is not just 5, 10, or 20 percent, but 5, 10 or 20 times more. Hundreds of percent more breast cancer, thousands of percent more prostate cancer are differences much greater than some of the differences found in an extensive study in China (The China Study, Campbell TC). Indians together make up one sixth of the world's population. They have the lowest cancer rates in the world. A reduced incidence of cancer cannot be the result of increased consumption of spices alone. Several dietary factors can contribute to India's low overall cancer rates. Besides the high consumption of herbs, Indians eat little (red) meat (holy cow) and 40 percent of the Indians are vegetarians. India is one of the largest producers and consumers of fresh fruits and vegetables. Indians also eat many other spices besides turmeric. Per weight unit, turmeric contains the highest content of antioxidants (Holt PR).

Omega-3 fish oil capsules, EPA and DHA have a beneficial effect on the heart and brain. Human brain cells are high in DHA. Sufficient fish in our menu is very important (Crawford MA 2012).

Benefits of Mediterranean food

The diet in Spain, Italy and Greece **is one of the healthiest eating habits in the world**. There are apparently fewer diseases here, and mortality from some chronic diseases is also less. This dietary pattern is rich in fruit, vegetables, fish, virgin olive oil and less saturated fat containing dairy products. Fats are necessary for the production of hormones and the absorption of the fat-soluble vitamins A, D and E. Olive oil gives food a taste and a feeling of satiety, so that you are less likely to get hungry again. This eating habit reduces the risk of cardiovascular disease, reduces the risk of diabetes, prolongs the lifespan and counts more healthy elderly people.

Avoid fast food and unhealthy trans fats

Fast food is in fashion. It is no longer rare for someone to go to bed with a bag of chips. Vegetable (unsaturated) fats are liquid at room temperature and can only be processed by the food industry as a solid substance. These fats are converted into partially hardened fat by a chemical process. Products that contain partially hydrogenated fats and trans fatty acids, such as margarine, chips, cookies, coffee milk powder, tarts, crackers and pizzas are bad for blood vessels.

So you become a hundred years

* do not fall

* do not have an accident

* don't get a cold

* do not choke, pneumonia most common cause of death for centenarians

How to stay healthy

* no colds

* don't smoke

* with clean indoor air, don't keep birds in home

* wash hands regularly

* eat more vegetable proteins

* do not eat animals

* train for one hour three times a week

Burning Belly Fat

Fat burning only starts after twenty minutes of exercise. Until this time of 20 minutes, especially carbohydrate reserves (the glycogen in the liver and muscles) are burned and you will not lose weight. This means that you start the fat burning process during the last part of the training. That is why it is better to exercise for one hour three times a week (3 x 40 minutes fat burning) than six times a week for half an hour (6 x 10 minutes fat burning). It does not matter what the training consists of. This can be brisk walking, slow jogging or a session on a treadmill or rowing machine.

SIMPLY MAKE YOUR OWN meals

Stick to this simple advice to get rid of excess body fat and prevent diseases. Only little whole meal bread, pasta and rice to lose weight faster. Nutrition must contain many vegetables, but also sufficient vegetable proteins and fats (fish, olive oil, avocado, etc.).

- *Start with a plant-based diet, and the need for animal proteins and fats will gradually decline*

In addition to diet, physical activity and extra antioxidant intake may counteract DNA methylation changes contributing to aging.

Fruit Breakfast

Start with two glasses of water

Oatmeal flakes with broken flax seed in soy yoghurt or soya light, almond milk or coconut milk, with fresh fruit. Like strawberries, raspberries, apples, pear, mandarin, orange, melon etc. Cut the fruit into pieces to preserve the dietary fiber.

Soup with the lunch

Make soup from vegetable broth. Think of tomato, vegetable, onion, pumpkin, mushroom, broccoli soup. A delicious soup can be made of all vegetables.

Salad with nuts, mushrooms, arugula, tomato, onion, garlic, green beans, kidney beans, chickpeas etc. Olive oil dressing.

Sandwich with salad of tuna, salmon, shrimp etc. or an omelet or hardboiled egg. Omega-3 rich fish such as salmon, herring, mackerel and shellfish like mussels are much healthier than red meat.

- *No sausages, hard-boiled eggs only, no meat (products) from the super, no insufficiently cooked BBQ meat, less dairy products, no raw milk cheese.*

Hot meal

Make especially use of herbs and spices. Replace the meat you were used to for example with chickpeas, brown or white beans. Make a delicious chili sin carne or curry dish with cauliflower, broccoli and chickpeas.

Bake and roast with coconut fat or olive oil

Coconut fat is very suitable for baking and roasting. Melt a coffee spoon (5 ml) in the pan is sufficient. When heating and roasting, less combustion products form than when heating the other vegetable oils, sunflower oil and olive oil.

No dessert

Avoid in case of excess weight sugars and quickly digestible carbohydrates. By sweetening, the liver chooses the path of least resistance (glycolysis) and provides the requested energy, glucose, and stores excess to body fat.

Drink black coffee with a little almond milk, green tea or ginger tea after the meal. Ginger tea can be made by cutting slices from ginger root and letting it boil in boiling water.

Olives, nuts.

- *Alcohol and wine in moderation. The degradation product acetaldehyde is harmful to our DNA. Too many wine acids damage the esophagus and stomach.*

The farm shop and local markets

Finally, it goes without saying that for our own health we can better stop the overproduction of animals for slaughter, pigs, chickens, eggs and their exports. A number of pig and chicken slaughterhouses can be closed if production is only allowed for domestic use. Farm shop and local markets are safer than oversized supermarkets. As farmers in France did, big chains like McDonald, Burger King and Kentucky Fried Chicken are better kept out now.

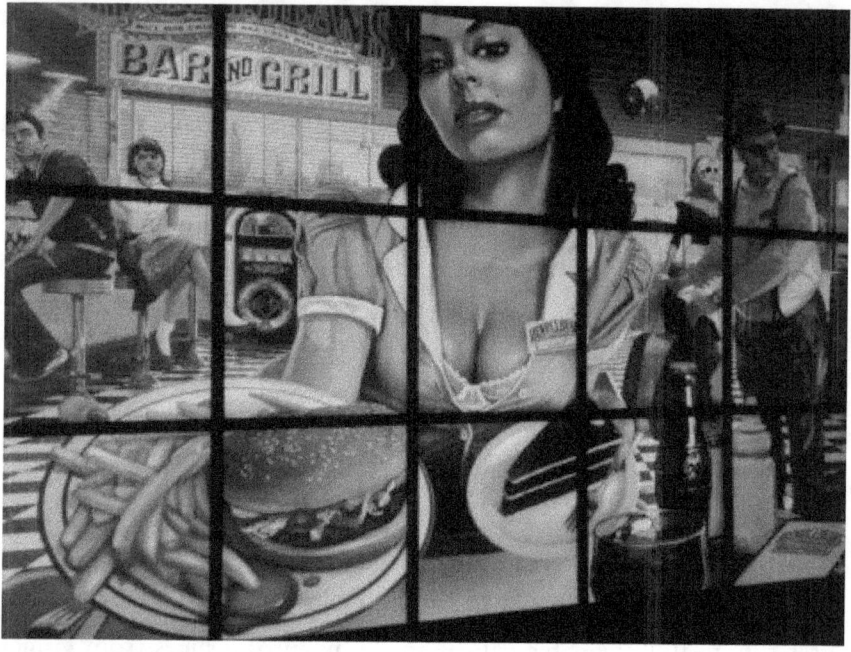

All the better restaurants nowadays also have a vegetarian menu. The farm shops could use a helping hand.

Vertical farming, multilayer cultivation

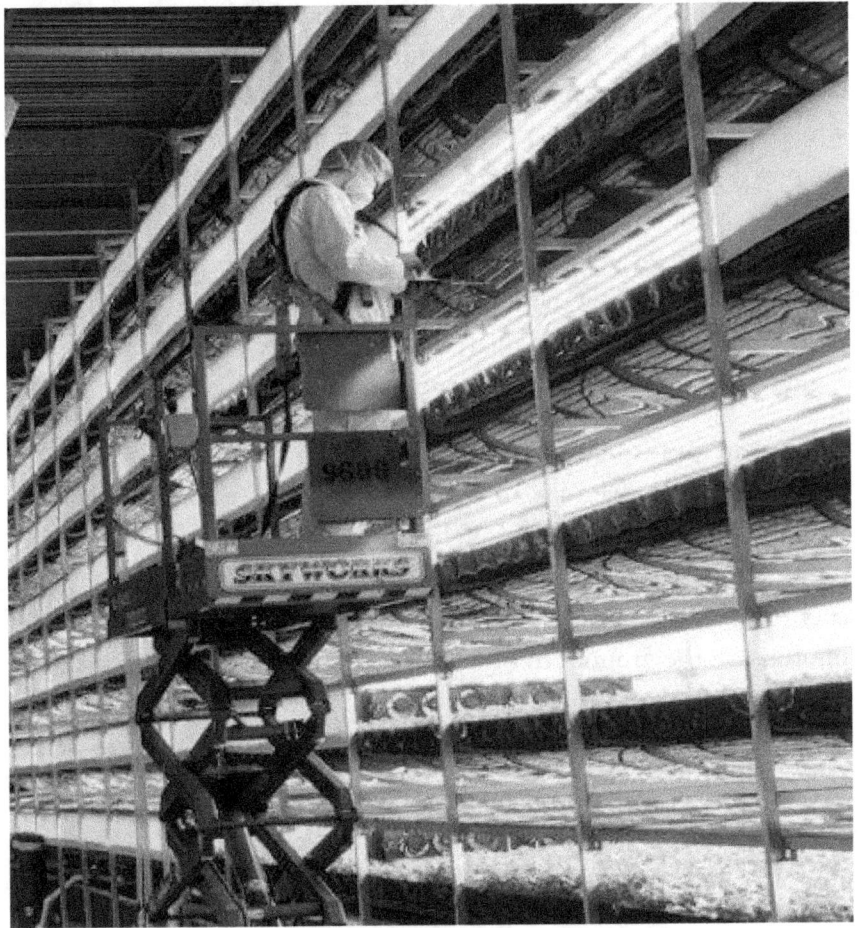

The usual agriculture and horticulture run on artificial fertilizers, pesticides and new plant varieties.

- Pesticides are no longer needed in such a closed system.
- Growing in two weeks which takes 30 days in the open

ground with 95 percent less water consumption, fewer fertilizers, and completely without pesticides.

Sunlight cannot be controlled. And the high-pressure sodium lamps with which Dutch growers provide extra light for their greenhouses can only be used to a limited extent. They give orange / yellow light and are too warm to place near plants. With the cooler LED lamps, which can contain all kinds of colors, engineers can develop a light recipe. They can choose the right combinations of wavelengths and light intensities, place the LED lamps near the plants, and opt for wider or narrower light beams. By altering the color of lights change the smell, taste and even the vitamin content of tomatoes. For more efficient growth, switch on the red light; to develop shorter plants with higher levels of antioxidants, use more blue light.

The reason for the higher yield, compared to greenhouses and outdoor cultivation, is that under LED lighting the entire plant, the whole year and long days can get enough light. In the uncontrolled sunlight, moreover, part is lost because one sheet gets too much and the other gets too little. Light is also lost due to reflection and the falling of photons on the ground. In order to make the collection of light more efficient, companies can drop light beams onto the leaves at certain angles. Or place LED lamps between plants. Strawberries are sweeter and tastier when the leaves and fruit are extra lighted. Dozens of vertical farms, also called 'vegetable factories' or 'indoor farms', supply spinach, bok choy, dill or cabbage every day. In climate-controlled rooms grow in four layers among others grow lettuce, strawberries, coriander and watercress. In an average Dutch greenhouse, the lettuce yield is 60 kilos per square meter of floor per year. 100 kilograms per square meter shelf will be taken in the vertical shelves. In Miyagi, Japan, a Japanese plant physiologist ordered 17,500 LED lamps that had to be installed in a former Sony factory. This factory supplies 10,000 unsprayed lettuce heads per day. In Singapore, Panasonic opened a fully automated indoor farm for 81 tons of vegetables every year. Aero Farms in Newark, USA, opened the largest so far, a nine-meter-high warehouse that will supply 250 different unsprayed vegetables and herbs.

Greenhouses are an area where machines are still surprisingly absent: picking crops such as tomatoes, peppers and strawberries has not yet been spent on robot hands on a large scale. Throughout the year, armies of pickers move into the greenhouses, which usually have relatively low wages and long and arduous working days. The picking robot is already used in Japan. In the absence of cheap labor, farmers there are in some cases satisfied with robots that harvest far less than human pickers. Even if the robot only harvests sixty or seventy percent of all strawberries, the grower earns more than if he hires relatively expensive pickers.

Agriculture on saline soils

- On Texel they succeeded in growing potatoes and vegetables on saline ground.
- Worldwide, 1.5 billion hectares of agricultural land are threatened by salinization. In areas where salinization poses the greatest threat, this offers a chance to feed families independently.
- Can the salty potato save people from the famine? Since 2010, Zilt Proefbedrijf Texel has been researching which crops grow on salty soil. Many species do well.
- The fermentation of seaweed releases 2/3 methane gas and 1/3 hydrogen gas which must only be collected and used better than the alternatives for natural gas that are currently available.

PUBLICATIONS AND BOOKS

Holst PAJ (1984) Bronchial carcinoma in bird keepers: an investigation in a general medical practice on a possible common relation.

Ned Tijdschr Geneeskd 128:899-902

Holst PAJ, Kromhout D, Brand R (1988) Pet birds as an independent risk for lung cancer.

Br Med J 297:1319-1321

Holst, PAJ (1991), Birdkeeping as a Source of Lung Cancer and Other Human Diseases. A Need for Higher Hygienic Standards.

Springer-Verlag ISBN 3-540-53555-1, Berlin/Heidelberg

Springer-Verlag ISBN 3-387-53555-1, New York

Kohlmeier L, Arminger A, Bartolomeycik S et al.(1992)

Pet birds as an independent risk for lung cancer: Case-control study.

Br Med J 305:986-989

Chu DJ, Guo SG, Pan CF, Wang J, Du Y, Lu XF, Yu ZY (2012) An experimental model for induction of lung cancer in rats by Chlamydia pneumoniae. Asian Pac J Cancer Prev. 2012;13(6):2819-22.

Chu DJ, Yao DE, Zhuang YF, Hong Y, Zhu XC, Fang ZR, Yu J and Yu ZY (2014) Azithromycin enhances the favorable results of paclitaxel and cisplatin in patients with advanced non-small cell lung cancer. Genet. Mol. Res. 13(2):2976-2805

Holst, PAJ (2014) The Last Chimpanzee, somewhere in the 21st century, the last chimpanzee will die, 2014 E-book APPLE

Paperback ISBN 978-94-02124-8-4

Holst, PAJ (2015) Plant-Based food is your Best Medicine

E-book APPLE 106 pages ISBN 9789082210569

Holst, PAJ (2016) Common Cancers are Zoonoses

E-book APPLE 197 pages ISBN 978-90-824963-3-8

Holst, PAJ (2016) Increase in Cancer is a Recent Event

E-book Apple ISBN 978-90-824963-0-7

Holst, PAJ (2016) PREVENTION IS BETTER THAN CURE

E-book 978-90-824963-2-1

Holst, PAJ (2019) Stop the Meatballs

Paperback 131 pages ISBN 978-1797658926

Holst, PAJ (2019) Our Inheritance from the Great Apes

Paperback. 146 pages ISBN 978-1081342159

Holst, PAJ (2019) Canimalism, E-book Kindle 119 pages

Paperback 120 pages Amazon.com ISBN 978-1694357762

Hardcover 120 pages Bravenewbooks.nl ISBN 978-9402198577

Consulted books

There is much scientific evidence published and also written in several books about health benefits of plant food for several diseases in later life. Change towards strictly plant-based foods is not easy. The image of the classic vegetarian complicates this transition. But read more about the health benefits to be achieved.

Forks Over Knives, the Plant-based Way to Health

Discusses the importance of eating a whole-foods, plant-based diet, describes how to transition to this type of diet, and provides one hundred twenty-five reci- pes for appetizers, soups, salads, main dishes, and desserts. Gene Stone & Campbell TC PhD

The China Study

Detailed study about the connection between nutrition and heart disease, diabetes, and cancer. The report also examines the source of nutritional confusion produced by powerful lobbies, government entities and opportunistic scientists. The China Study observed whether there were patterns of associations for different dietary, lifestyle and disease characteristics within the survey of 65 counties, 130 villages and 6,500 adults and their families. **Campbell TC**, Campbell TM (2006) **The China Study.** electronic Book Apple

How Not to Die

The vast majority of premature deaths can be prevented through simple changes in diet and lifestyle. In How Not to Die, Dr. Michael Greger, the internationally renowned nutrition expert, physician, and founder of NutritionFacts.org, examines the fifteen top causes of premature death in America-heart disease, various cancers, diabetes, Parkinson's, high blood pressure, and more-and explains how nutritional and lifestyle interventions can trump prescription pills and pharmaceutical and surgical approaches, freeing us to live healthier lives. Gene Stone & Michael Greger MD

Proteinaholic, how Our Obsession with Meat is Killing Us and What We Can Do About it

Whether you are seeing a doctor, nutritionist, or a trainer, all of them advise to eat more protein. Foods, drinks, and supplements are loaded with extra protein. Many people use protein for weight control, to gain or lose pounds, while others believe it gives them more energy and is essential for a longer, healthier life. Now, Dr. Garth Davis, an expert in weight loss asks, is all this protein making us healthier? The answer, he emphatically argues, is NO. Too much protein is actually making us sick, fat, and tired, according to Dr. Davis. The healthiest countries in the world eat far less protein than we do and yet we have an entire nation on a protein binge getting sicker by the day. Garth Davis MD & Howard Jacobson

Guns, Germs, and Steel: The Fates of Human Societies

Guns, Germs, and Steel seek to answer the biggest question of post-Ice-Age human history: why Eurasian peoples, rather than peoples of other continents, became the ones to develop the ingredients of power (guns, germs, and steel) and to expand around the world. Africans enjoyed a huge head start, because Africa is the continent with by far the longest history of human occupation. North America is a big fertile continent, with the result that it supports the richest and most productive nation today. Australia provides by far the earliest evidence for human ability to cross wide water gaps, and some of the earliest widespread evidence for behaviorally modern humans. Why, nevertheless, were Eurasians the ones to expand? The reasons were continental differences in the available wild plant and animal species suitable for domestication, resulting in earlier domestication of a more productive suite of domesticates in Eurasia, plus Eurasia's east/west axis that facilitated the spread of those domesticates throughout Eurasia. Europeans were able to spread at the expense of other peoples by infecting them (usually unintentionally) with epidemic infectious diseases such as smallpox and measles, to which Europeans had evolved some genetic resistance and had acquired much immune (antibody-based) resistance through historical and lifetime exposure respectively, while unexposed non-European peoples had no such exposure, hence no such resistance. The exchange of major epidemic infectious diseases was one-sided, because most of those diseases in the temperate zones came to us humans from diseases of our domestic animals (such as cattle, pigs, and chickens) with which our ancestors lived in close contact after those animal species had been domesticated. But of the world's 14 species of valuable domestic mammals, 13 were Eurasian, only one American, and none Australian. Hence Eurasians ended up as disease bearers, and with much resistance themselves to their own diseases. Jared Diamond 1997.

Dead Zone, where the wild things were

A tour of some of the world's most iconic and endangered species, and what we can do to save them. Climate change and habitat destruction are not the only culprits behind so many animals facing extinction. The impact of consumer demand for cheap meat is equally devastating and it is vital that we confront this problem if we are to stand a chance of reducing its effect on the world around us. We are falsely led to believe that squeezing animals into factory farms and cultivating crops in vast, chemical-soaked prairies is a necessary evil, an efficient means of providing for an ever- expanding global population while leaving land free for wildlife. Our planet's resources are reaching breaking point: awareness is slowly building that the wellbeing of society depends on a thriving natural world.

Large amounts of nitrogen from fertilizer and manure are distributed annually over agricultural land. No doubt that it increases crop yield, but plants do not absorb it completely, so that more fertilizer and animal waste is added than the plants need. Only a fraction of what is applied to the soil ends up in the crops. The rest flows to our rivers. Nitrogen and phosphorus levels, dead organisms are increasing in the Gulf of Mexico, the Rhône Delta, the North Sea, the Baltic Sea and the Adriatic Sea. Oxygen levels fall in these coastal waters. From the author of the internationally acclaimed **Farmageddon.** Dead Zone takes us on an eye-opening investigative journey across the globe, focussing on a dozen iconic species one-by-one and looking in each case at the role that industrial farming is playing in their plight. This is a passionate wake-up call for us all, laying bare the myths that prop up factory farming before exploring what we can do to save the planet with healthy food. Phillip Lymbery. 2017

David Attenborrough - A Life on Our Planet

Hundreds of studies around the world have confirmed that something is going on. The consequences will be more far-reaching than the pollution of the soil and water in a few countries that are unlucky enough to be caused by explosions at a nuclear power station. Ultimately, this could lead to the disruption and collapse of everything we rely on.

This is the real tragedy of our time: the accelerating decline in the biodiversity of our planet. We need overwhelming biodiversity if life on our planet is really to flourish. Only when billions of different individual organisms make the best use of all the resources and opportunities they encounter, and when millions of species live interlinked lives that are interlinked in such a way that they sustain each other, can the planet function smoothly. The greater the biodiversity of our planet, the safer all life on earth, including ourselves, will be. However, biodiversity is plunging under the influence of our current way of life.

We lead our pleasant lives in the shadow of a disaster that we ourselves are causing. This catastrophe is caused by the very things that enable us to create an atmosphere of well-being. And it is logical that we will continue to do so until we have a decisive reason to stop doing so, and an appealing alternative. The natural world is in decline. The evidence is convincing it will lead to our destruction. There is another alternative to turn the tide for the better, if we act now. Part of the solution may well be in the Netherlands, one of the few countries explicitly mentioned in the film. Attenborough explains that it is a densely populated country, but it is still the world's second largest exporter of food. There is no mention of the fact that a large proportion of these exports also involve meat and dairy products.

Attenborough shows the efficient way in which vegetables are grown in our country, in greenhouses and under artificial sunlight. That is the future, he thinks. I don't want to be too praiseworthy, but your skills are an example to many of us", explains the naturalist when asked. He also points out how the Netherlands deals with seawater. One of the problems we are going to have to deal with as a result of climate change is flooding cities. You can teach the rest of the world a lot about that too".

Acknowledgement

F or the bachelor examination I did my pathology exam with Professor Dr. A. de Minjer. My thesis on small cell lung cancer was discussed and the Minjer took me to the pottery museum where they stopped for some time in front of a preparation with lung carcinoma of a smoker. De Minjer pointed that lung cancer and breast cancer for the coming years would be the biggest challenges of medicine. More than fifty years later, that is still the case.

Because of the many consultation hours and home visits, ten lung cancer patients came to my attention in the general practice. Of these, there were six bird keepers in the years before diagnosis. After consulting with professor F. de Waard of the RIVM, department of epidemiology, I have set up a ten-year practice survey and follow-up studies. The statistical link was demonstrated, later confirmed in studies in Berlin and Glasgow.

I would like to thank professor Peernel Zwart (Department of Veterinary Pathology, Division for Diseases of Special Animals. State University

Utrecht, Head: Prof. Dr. P. ZWART) for his comments after the presentation of my research findings. "Original ideas and observations are rare. They are especially valuable if checked in practice, critically evaluated and supported by material independently collected by others. It is to the very personal credit of Dr. P.A.J. Holst that he noticed a potential connection between the keeping of birds and the occurrence of lung cancer among members of households where they are kept. He has pursued the idea in his private practice and over 12 years kept records of every single patient. The data were critically and statistically analyzed and supplemented by data and materials collected by lung specialists".

Research in cancer, especially in lung cancer in humans, has involved a large input of science and has contributed considerable to knowledge of the many factors involved. A new aspect is presented in avian products, spread in the house in the form of fine dust particles, inhaled deeply, cause irritation and contribute to local immune responses in the lungs. Much later, in 2012, laboratory experiments proved the link between lung cancer and Chlamydia pneumonia infection (Chu DJ 2012 & 2014).

I was impressed by Dr. Michael Greger's publications "Emergence and Resurgence of Zoonotic Infectious Diseases".

I would like to thank Eleonora van het Groenewout for her critical reading of the manuscript and advice on the layout. I also thank Paul Boute for his philosophical reflection on the struggle of the zoonoses as David against Goliath.

Finally, I would like to thank Rob Hamers, who is an expert in phytotherapy, for his critical comments and contribution in the field of lifestyle medicine.

Author biography

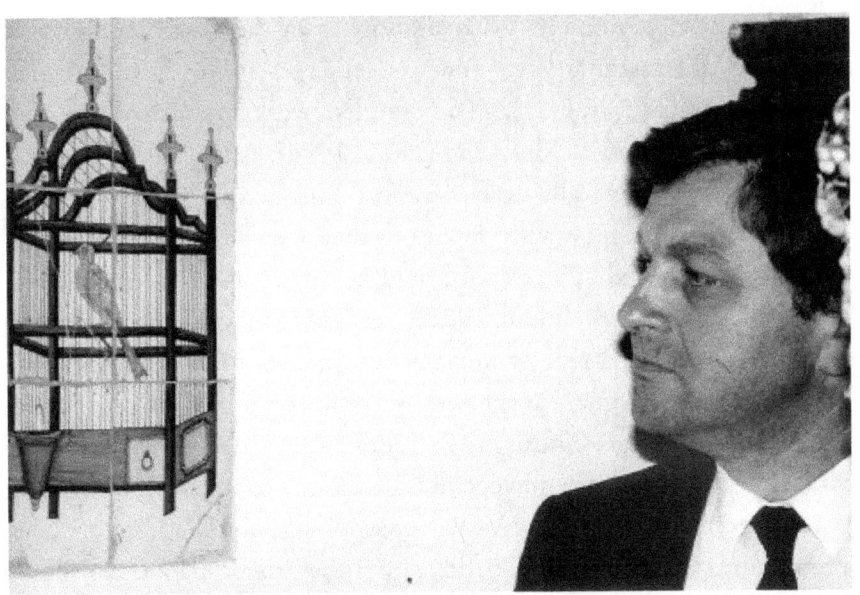

Dr. Peter Holst worked until 1984 as a general practitioner in The Hague area, the Netherlands. As a starting general practitioner in 1970 he saw a young girl with a severe case of Chlamydia pneumonia. After treatment with antibiotics she recovered. Because she kept a budgie in a cage in her bedroom, he assumed "the presence of a caged bird at home could be responsible for more serious disease". In his practice he also treated a 17 year old boy with an osteosarcoma in his upper leg, where he died from. As a hobby he kept and bred about 100 tropical birds in a basement room.

Because of the many consultation hours and home visits, ten lung cancer patients came to his attention in the following years. Of these, there were six bird keepers in the years before diagnosis.

After consulting a professor in the epidemioly he started a ten-year practice-survey. He did his research with the University of Utrecht. Unique by the combination of veterinary and human medicine. Diseases that from animals to humans can pass (zoonoses) are becoming more common. With support from the Dutch Prevention Fund, he did research into new cancer cases in his own practice (ten-year practice survey). The results were published in the Netherlands Journal of Medicine (Holst 1984). After this he began a case-control study of all newly diagnosed lung cancer patients in all hospitals of The Hague with the aid of their own lung specialists. The results of these studies were published in the British Medical Journal (Holst, Kromhout & Brand 1988). Bird keeping and bird breeding were proven to be a risk of lung cancer. In the study of lung cancer patients in The Hague, except the risk of keeping birds in the house, especially breeding of birds, they found also a decreased intake of vitamin C. Fresh fruits and vegetables are eaten too little. During long sea voyages in the era of the VOC (East India Company), sailors died prematurely from vitamin C deficiency. Today, the fast-food consumer get food from around the world on his plate. Pigs, cattle and chickens are fed with fish meal and soybean meal from South America. Fresh fruits and vegetables are eaten too little.

With the Dutch Organization for Applied Scientific Research (TNO Delft) he then carried out dust measurements in homes of bird keepers.

In 1987, this research led to his PhD at the University of Utrecht on the relationship he demonstrated between breeding and keeping birds indoors and lung cancer. He defended the hypothesis that lung cancer in bird keepers and bird breeders is the result of persistent infection of the deeper basal cells in the airways. These basal cells are still multipotent and do not die if the cell is infected with a bacterium like the Chlamydia that can only propagate in a living host cell. His promoters were prof. F. de Waard, epidemiologist of the RIVM, professor P. Zwart, head of the special veterinary faculty University Utrecht and D. Kromhout, nutritional epidemiologist. The practical studies and the dust measurements with TNO were supported by the Dutch Prevention Fund.

Holst specialized from 1984 in Occupational and Environmental Health Services. Some years from its founding in 1991, he was a member of the International Society of Indoor Air Quality (ISIAQ). He has published in various medical journals and has written books on indoor air hygiene and preventive medicine.

In 2012 a laboratory experiment proved the link between lung cancer and Chlamydia pneumonia infection.

His interest in the link between breeding tropical birds and cancer has expanded to the health risks of the intensive rearing of poultry, pigs and cattle for consumption. Since the fifties of the 20th century, artificial breeding in livestock has increased sharply. In the past fifty years, our diet has become increasingly unnatural. More meat products from animals, solely bred for consumption, cause more chronic diseases. An increase that keeps pace with the recent increase in cancer mortality.